THE TEACHINGS OF *Joshua*

The Joshua Diet
Playbook

VOLUME I

Week 1 to Week 13

Printed in the United States of America

First Printing, 2016

ISBN-13: 978-1541078666

ISBN: 1541078667

Week 1 to week 13

Transformation begins with the first act of inspiration. You were inspired to purchase this playbook. When you act upon inspiration from a high emotional state of being, you can trust that the action will lead you closer to your desire. So, we ask you now, what is your desire? Is your desire to sculpt a lean and healthy body? That is a wonderful idea, but you must dig a little deeper than that. Why do you want to change the look and feel of your body? What is the motivation behind it? Do you feel a lean body will solve any problem? It will not. Do you believe a lean body will make you happy? It will not.

Your body is simply a reflection of how you feel about yourself up until this very point in time. You must feel better now and your body will reflect how you feel. You must be happy in your body now and your body will make you happy. If you feel sad, your body will be your excuse to feeling sad. Feel better and you will be inspired to do things that align with how you feel.

So we ask you to intentionally and consciously decide why you want a lean and healthy body. There is a good answer and here it is:

"I want a lean and healthy body because I want to feel what that is like. I want to experience the feeling of optimal health and well-being. I want to feel the joy of being comfortable in my body. I want to enjoy the ease of living in optimal health. I want to feel good and I want to feel good in my body!"

This is the first step in a thirteen week journey of improvement. There are no rules. There are no goals. There are no measurements of any kind. There is no way to compare yourself to any standard. You will not be interested in the successes of others for there is no way to judge others' success. Just by making the decision to embark on this journey, you have made a bold statement to the universe. You are interested in pursuing a fun and exciting idea. What would it be like to immerse yourself in a program that is focused on making you feel better?

You are not to be attached to results, all you are interested in doing is filling out each line in every page of this playbook. This is not work, this is intended to be play. These exercises are meant to be fun. It is up to you to make it fun. It is your choice to make it work or play. You choose the perspective. You choose to do the exercises or not. Like everything else in life, you are in charge of what happens next.

If you play along with us, we will promise you this: your life will be forever changed. Will you be able to create a body as lean as a supermodel's? We aren't sure if that is really even a goal to consider. Will your body return to optimal health and well-being? Maybe it will and maybe not. We can't tell you what will happen for you because you are unique. What we can promise is that by the end of this first playbook, your set of beliefs will be vastly improved. You will have many more beneficial beliefs. You will have a radically different thought process. You will be much more in control of your thoughts. Your approach to life will be transformed. And as a result of all this, your reality will shift and reflect your new and improved set of beliefs. Your vibration will be forever raised and your life will look much brighter and more promising.

There's nothing you need to do but to feel good. In feeling good and focusing on your desire (because you want the feeling of the desire and no other reason), you will be given inspiration to act. You are unique. There is no one on earth like you. There is no diet or exercise routine that works for everyone. You will be guided to what works for you. It may not happen tomorrow or this week, but inspiration will come. You received inspiration to start this program and you will receive the inspiration for each and every step along the way.

Give up your attachments. Give up your attachment to a target weight. Give up your attachment to a perfect shape. Do not ever compare yourself unfavorably to anyone else. Compare yourself to you. In one month, compare yourself to how you felt when you started. In thirteen weeks, compare how you feel then to how you felt today. That's how you'll know you made progress. That's how you can tell that you've succeeded.

This is not a thirteen week journey, this is a life-long approach to life. You start here. As you complete each day, you build momentum. In time, it will get easier and easier. If you have not meditated before, you will come to enjoy it and look forward to it. Everything will become routine. As you practice meditation, setting intentions, writing lists of appreciation and gratitude, writing affirmations, and conducting experiments, you will gradually move into a new approach to life and you'll start to see things differently. Your life will begin to look new and fresh and the things you once thought were important or scary will fade away.

There is another approach to life. The life you have lived up until this moment has unfolded perfectly to bring you here. You are at the perfect starting point. We can see the path ahead of you, but unfortunately you cannot. It is easy. Nothing should be hard. If it's difficult, don't do it. If it's not enjoyable, try something else. You will find what is right for you. It will get easier. It does not have to be hard. Trust us when we say "It's all downhill from here."

You are loved more than you can imagine by more than you could ever count,

We are Joshua

QUOTE OF THE DAY:

❝ The only way to manifesting the slim, strong and lean body you want is by first achieving a healthy and fit mind." *Joshua*

Morning Playbook

MEDITATION:

Duration .... Type..

Time of Day .... Satisfaction Level: 1 2 3 4 5 6 7 8 9 10

Notes: ....

....

APPRECIATION:

List 3 things you appreciate about your life:

1. ....

   ....

2. ....

   ....

3. ....

   ....

INTENTIONS:

Set your general intentions for the day:

....

....

....

....

....

....

....

....

Evening Playbook

GRATITUDE:

List 3 things you are grateful for (which can include future manifestations):

1. ....

....

2. ....

....

3. ....

....

AFFIRMATIONS:

Write 3 affirmations:

1. ....

....

2. ....

....

3. ....

....

FEELINGS:

How did you feel today? ....

How do you feel now? ....

How do you intend to feel tomorrow? ....

INSPIRATION:

Did you receive inspiration today? ....

Describe what you were inspired to do or say ....

....

FOOD EXPERIMENT:

What single item of food did you experiment with today?...............

Describe how you felt? ....

....

Does your unique body process this food easily? ....

QUOTE OF THE DAY:

" There is one way to maintain your body and one way only; through the power of your mind. Until you've trained your mind how to think, you cannot expect the long-term results you desire. It all has to do with the thoughts that enter your head and how you choose to deal with them." *Joshua*

Morning Playbook

MEDITATION:

Duration .... Type...

Time of Day .... Satisfaction Level: 1 2 3 4 5 6 7 8 9 10

Notes: ....
....

APPRECIATION:

List 3 things you appreciate about your life:

1. ....
   ....
2. ....
   ....
3. ....
   ....

INTENTIONS:

Set your general intentions for the day:

....
....
....
....
....
....
....

Evening Playbook

GRATITUDE:

List 3 things you are grateful for (which can include future manifestations):

1. ....

....

2. ....

....

3. ....

....

AFFIRMATIONS:

Write 3 affirmations:

1. ....

....

2. ....

....

3. ....

....

FEELINGS:

How did you feel today?...

How do you feel now? ....

How do you intend to feel tomorrow? ....

INSPIRATION:

Did you receive inspiration today? ....

Describe what you were inspired to do or say ....

....

FOOD EXPERIMENT:

What single item of food did you experiment with today?...............................

Describe how you felt? ....

....

Does your unique body process this food easily? ....

QUOTE OF THE DAY:

 A healthy mind will be able to overcome the requests of the body." *Joshua*

Morning Playbook

MEDITATION:

Duration .... Type..

Time of Day .... Satisfaction Level: 1 2 3 4 5 6 7 8 9 10

Notes: ....

....

....

APPRECIATION:

List 3 things you appreciate about your life:

1. ....

....

2. ....

....

3. ....

....

INTENTIONS:

Set your general intentions for the day:

....

....

....

....

....

....

....

....

Evening Playbook

List 3 things you are grateful for (which can include future manifestations):

1. ....
   ....

2. ....
   ....

3. ....
   ....

AFFIRMATIONS:

Write 3 affirmations:

1. ....
   ....

2. ....
   ....

3. ....
   ....

FEELINGS:

How did you feel today? ....

How do you feel now? ....

How do you intend to feel tomorrow? ....

INSPIRATION:

Did you receive inspiration today? ....

Describe what you were inspired to do or say ....
....

FOOD EXPERIMENT:

What single item of food did you experiment with today? ....

Describe how you felt? ....
....

Does your unique body process this food easily? ....

QUOTE OF THE DAY:

" As you change your vibration, you create an environment where you allow yourself to receive inspiration. This inspiration is crucial to losing weight. You must feel inspired. You must act in accordance with that inspiration. As you raise your vibration, allow inspiration to come, and adjust your attitude, you attract thoughts, feelings, beliefs, and actions that align with what is wanted." *Joshua*

Morning Playbook

MEDITATION:

Duration .... Type...

Time of Day .... Satisfaction Level: 1 2 3 4 5 6 7 8 9 10

Notes: ....

....

APPRECIATION:

List 3 things you appreciate about your life:

1. ....

....

2. ....

....

3. ....

....

INTENTIONS:

Set your general intentions for the day:

....

....

....

....

....

....

....

Evening Playbook

GRATITUDE:

List 3 things you are grateful for (which can include future manifestations):

1. ....
....
2. ....
....
3. ....
....

AFFIRMATIONS:

Write 3 affirmations:

1. ....
....
2. ....
....
3. ....
....

FEELINGS:

How did you feel today? ....

How do you feel now? ....

How do you intend to feel tomorrow? ....

INSPIRATION:

Did you receive inspiration today? ....

Describe what you were inspired to do or say ....
....

FOOD EXPERIMENT:

What single item of food did you experiment with today? ....

Describe how you felt? ....
....

Does your unique body process this food easily? ....

QUOTE OF THE DAY:

" If you can maintain your focus on how you feel, you can adjust your emotional state at anytime simply by being aware of those times when you feel a dip, realizing that your tendency will be to reach for outside fixes, realize that the thoughts that are flowing to you have been attracted by your state of being, and understand that you have the ability to reach for better-feeling thoughts." *Joshua*

Morning Playbook

MEDITATION:

Duration ....   Type...

Time of Day ....   Satisfaction Level: 1   2   3   4   5   6   7   8   9   10

Notes: ....

....

APPRECIATION:

List 3 things you appreciate about your life:

1. ....

....

2. ....

....

3. ....

....

INTENTIONS:

Set your general intentions for the day:

....

....

....

....

....

....

....

Evening Playbook

GRATITUDE:

List 3 things you are grateful for (which can include future manifestations):

1. ....

   ....

2. ....

   ....

3. ....

   ....

AFFIRMATIONS:

Write 3 affirmations:

1. ....

   ....

2. ....

   ....

3. ....

   ....

FEELINGS:

How did you feel today? ....

How do you feel now? ....

How do you intend to feel tomorrow? ....

INSPIRATION:

Did you receive inspiration today? ....

Describe what you were inspired to do or say ....

....

FOOD EXPERIMENT:

What single item of food did you experiment with today?....................

Describe how you felt? ....

....

Does your unique body process this food easily? ....

QUOTE OF THE DAY:

" There is nothing you need to do to create the body you desire other than building the most important muscle in your body; your brain." *Joshua*

Morning Playbook

MEDITATION:

Duration ....   Type...

Time of Day ....   Satisfaction Level: 1   2   3   4   5   6   7   8   9   10

Notes: ....
....
....

APPRECIATION:

List 3 things you appreciate about your life:

1. ....
   ....

2. ....
   ....

3. ....
   ....

INTENTIONS:

Set your general intentions for the day:

....
....
....
....
....
....
....

Evening Playbook

GRATITUDE:

List 3 things you are grateful for (which can include future manifestations):

1. ....
....

2. ....
....

3. ....
....

AFFIRMATIONS:

Write 3 affirmations:

1. ....
....

2. ....
....

3. ....
....

FEELINGS:

How did you feel today? ....

How do you feel now? ....

How do you intend to feel tomorrow? ....

INSPIRATION:

Did you receive inspiration today? ....

Describe what you were inspired to do or say ....
....

FOOD EXPERIMENT:

What single item of food did you experiment with today?..........................

Describe how you felt? ....
....

Does your unique body process this food easily? ....

QUOTE OF THE DAY:

" If you loved yourself, if you felt confident and worthy, if you were secure, if you approached life from a stance that everything is right as it is, if you were non-resistant, you would be free from all stress and you would maintain a weight which is ideal for your body." *Joshua*

Morning Playbook

MEDITATION:

Duration ....   Type...

Time of Day ....   Satisfaction Level: 1   2   3   4   5   6   7   8   9   10

Notes: ....

....

APPRECIATION:

List 3 things you appreciate about your life:

1. ....

....

2. ....

....

3. ....

....

INTENTIONS:

Set your general intentions for the day:

....

....

....

....

....

....

....

Evening Playbook

GRATITUDE:

List 3 things you are grateful for (which can include future manifestations):

1. ....
....

2. ....
....

3. ....
....

AFFIRMATIONS:

Write 3 affirmations:

1. ....
....

2. ....
....

3. ....
....

FEELINGS:

How did you feel today? ....

How do you feel now? ....

How do you intend to feel tomorrow? ....

INSPIRATION:

Did you receive inspiration today? ....

Describe what you were inspired to do or say ....
....

FOOD EXPERIMENT:

What single item of food did you experiment with today?.....................

Describe how you felt? ....
....

Does your unique body process this food easily? ....

QUOTE OF THE DAY:

66 Fat cells want to feel good too. Fat cells have a reason for being. Fat cells would like to continue to provide benefit for the body. Fat cells want to be useful. Fat cells want to be burned as fuel. Fat is extremely good as a form of energy storage. Burn the fat and you'll feel good because your body will be working as it should. Hate the fat and you cause the body to behave in contrast to how it was designed." *Joshua*

Morning Playbook

MEDITATION:

Duration ....   Type...

Time of Day ....   Satisfaction Level: 1   2   3   4   5   6   7   8   9   10

Notes: ....

....

APPRECIATION:

List 3 things you appreciate about your life:

1. ....

....

2. ....

....

3. ....

....

INTENTIONS:

Set your general intentions for the day:

....

....

....

....

....

....

Evening Playbook

GRATITUDE:

List 3 things you are grateful for (which can include future manifestations):

1. ....

   ....

2. ....

   ....

3. ....

   ....

AFFIRMATIONS:

Write 3 affirmations:

1. ....

   ....

2. ....

   ....

3. ....

   ....

FEELINGS:

How did you feel today? ....

How do you feel now? ....

How do you intend to feel tomorrow? ....

INSPIRATION:

Did you receive inspiration today? ....

Describe what you were inspired to do or say ....

....

FOOD EXPERIMENT:

What single item of food did you experiment with today?.................

Describe how you felt? ....

....

Does your unique body process this food easily? ....

QUOTE OF THE DAY:

" What is in your life now perfectly matches your vibration. Most of it is very, very good, but there are some things you may wish to change. In order for these things to change, your vibration must change first." *Joshua*

Morning Playbook

MEDITATION:

Duration .... Type...

Time of Day .... Satisfaction Level: 1 2 3 4 5 6 7 8 9 10

Notes: ....

....

APPRECIATION:

List 3 things you appreciate about your life:

1. ....

....

2. ....

....

3. ....

....

INTENTIONS:

Set your general intentions for the day:

....

....

....

....

....

....

Evening Playbook

GRATITUDE:

List 3 things you are grateful for (which can include future manifestations):

1. ....

   ....

2. ....

   ....

3. ....

   ....

AFFIRMATIONS:

Write 3 affirmations:

1. ....

   ....

2. ....

   ....

3. ....

   ....

FEELINGS:

How did you feel today? ....

How do you feel now? ....

How do you intend to feel tomorrow? ....

INSPIRATION:

Did you receive inspiration today? ....

Describe what you were inspired to do or say ....

....

FOOD EXPERIMENT:

What single item of food did you experiment with today? ....

Describe how you felt? ....

....

Does your unique body process this food easily? ....

QUOTE OF THE DAY:

" Feeling good is the only thing that really matters. This is a feeling reality. All you're ever doing in any moment is feeling. You're either feeling good, content, pleasant, happy, secure, etc. or your feeling bad, scared, worried, insecure, bored, etc. Strive to feel good." *Joshua*

Morning Playbook

MEDITATION:

Duration .... Type..

Time of Day .... Satisfaction Level: 1 2 3 4 5 6 7 8 9 10

Notes: ....
....

APPRECIATION:

List 3 things you appreciate about your life:

1. ....
....

2. ....
....

3. ....
....

INTENTIONS:

Set your general intentions for the day:

....
....
....
....
....
....

Evening Playbook

GRATITUDE:

List 3 things you are grateful for (which can include future manifestations):

1. ....
   ....

2. ....
   ....

3. ....
   ....

AFFIRMATIONS:

Write 3 affirmations:

1. ....
   ....

2. ....
   ....

3. ....
   ....

FEELINGS:

How did you feel today? ....

How do you feel now? ....

How do you intend to feel tomorrow? ....

INSPIRATION:

Did you receive inspiration today? ....

Describe what you were inspired to do or say ....
....

FOOD EXPERIMENT:

What single item of food did you experiment with today?.................................

Describe how you felt? ....
....

Does your unique body process this food easily? ....

QUOTE OF THE DAY:

❝ When you strive to feel good, when you intend to feel good, you set forth powerful energies out into the universe. The universe yields to how you feel. When you feel strong, confident, loving, happy, funny, exuberant, etc. the universe must bring you evidence of how you are feeling. You will encounter more fun, more love, more satisfaction, more success and more moments that reinforce your good feelings. It is just the design of the system." *Joshua*

Morning Playbook

MEDITATION:

Duration ....   Type..

Time of Day ....   Satisfaction Level: 1   2   3   4   5   6   7   8   9   10

Notes: ....

....

APPRECIATION:

List 3 things you appreciate about your life:

1. ....

   ....

2. ....

   ....

3. ....

   ....

INTENTIONS:

Set your general intentions for the day:

....

....

....

....

....

....

Evening Playbook

GRATITUDE:

List 3 things you are grateful for (which can include future manifestations):

1. ....
   ....

2. ....
   ....

3. ....
   ....

AFFIRMATIONS:

Write 3 affirmations:

1. ....
   ....

2. ....
   ....

3. ....
   ....

FEELINGS:

How did you feel today? ....

How do you feel now? ....

How do you intend to feel tomorrow? ....

INSPIRATION:

Did you receive inspiration today? ....

Describe what you were inspired to do or say ....
....

FOOD EXPERIMENT:

What single item of food did you experiment with today? ....

Describe how you felt? ....
....

Does your unique body process this food easily? ....

QUOTE OF THE DAY:

" Feel good now and you will attract a body that also feels good." *Joshua*

Morning Playbook

MEDITATION:

Duration .... Type...

Time of Day .... Satisfaction Level: 1 2 3 4 5 6 7 8 9 10

Notes: ....

....

....

APPRECIATION:

List 3 things you appreciate about your life:

1. ....

  ....

2. ....

  ....

3. ....

  ....

INTENTIONS:

Set your general intentions for the day:

....

....

....

....

....

....

....

Evening Playbook

GRATITUDE:

List 3 things you are grateful for (which can include future manifestations):

1. ....
....

2. ....
....

3. ....
....

AFFIRMATIONS:

Write 3 affirmations:

1. ....
....

2. ....
....

3. ....
....

FEELINGS:

How did you feel today? ....

How do you feel now? ....

How do you intend to feel tomorrow? ....

INSPIRATION:

Did you receive inspiration today? ....

Describe what you were inspired to do or say ....
....

FOOD EXPERIMENT:

What single item of food did you experiment with today?..

Describe how you felt? ....
....

Does your unique body process this food easily? ....

QUOTE OF THE DAY:

66 By focusing on what is not wanted - excess weight - you bring more of it into your reality. It is simply the primary law of the universe at work." *Joshua*

Morning Playbook

MEDITATION:

Duration ....   Type..

Time of Day ....   Satisfaction Level: 1 2 3 4 5 6 7 8 9 10

Notes: ....

....

....

APPRECIATION:

List 3 things you appreciate about your life:

1. ....

   ....

2. ....

   ....

3. ....

   ....

INTENTIONS:

Set your general intentions for the day:

....

....

....

....

....

....

....

Evening Playbook

GRATITUDE:

List 3 things you are grateful for (which can include future manifestations):

1. ....

....

2. ....

....

3. ....

....

AFFIRMATIONS:

Write 3 affirmations:

1. ....

....

2. ....

....

3. ....

....

FEELINGS:

How did you feel today? ....

How do you feel now? ....

How do you intend to feel tomorrow? ....

INSPIRATION:

Did you receive inspiration today? ....

Describe what you were inspired to do or say ....

....

FOOD EXPERIMENT:

What single item of food did you experiment with today?........................

Describe how you felt? ....

....

Does your unique body process this food easily? ....

QUOTE OF THE DAY:

" You have the ability to choose any thought and you also have the ability to choose any belief. Beliefs are not made in stone. They are illusions. Most of your beliefs have never really been tested. You carry with you a set of beliefs based on chance encounters and what other people have told you. Since they've been with you a long, long time, they've gained momentum. You believe your beliefs are true, but most are not. Now is the time to challenge your limiting beliefs and shore up your beneficial beliefs." *Joshua*

Morning Playbook

MEDITATION:

Duration .... Type...

Time of Day .... Satisfaction Level: 1 2 3 4 5 6 7 8 9 10

Notes: ....

....

APPRECIATION:

List 3 things you appreciate about your life:

1. ....

   ....

2. ....

   ....

3. ....

   ....

INTENTIONS:

Set your general intentions for the day:

....

....

....

....

....

Evening Playbook

GRATITUDE:

List 3 things you are grateful for (which can include future manifestations):

1. ....
....
2. ....
....
3. ....
....

AFFIRMATIONS:

Write 3 affirmations:

1. ....
....
2. ....
....
3. ....
....

FEELINGS:

How did you feel today? ....

How do you feel now? ....

How do you intend to feel tomorrow? ....

INSPIRATION:

Did you receive inspiration today? ....

Describe what you were inspired to do or say ....
....

FOOD EXPERIMENT:

What single item of food did you experiment with today?...........................

Describe how you felt? ....
....

Does your unique body process this food easily? ....

QUOTE OF THE DAY:

" When you encounter any negative emotion, this is a manifestation event which is attempting to change some limiting belief. Since negative emotion is an unpleasant feeling, these events often feel unpleasant. You will think that something bad has happened. However, nothing bad has happened, it's just that from your perspective, you are encountering something that scares you and negative emotion arises to alert you to this irrational fear. There is some limiting belief based in an irrational fear which causes you to feel negative emotion." *Joshua*

Morning Playbook

MEDITATION:

Duration ....   Type..

Time of Day ....   Satisfaction Level: 1   2   3   4   5   6   7   8   9   10

Notes: ....

....

APPRECIATION:

List 3 things you appreciate about your life:

1. ....

....

2. ....

....

3. ....

....

INTENTIONS:

Set your general intentions for the day:

....

....

....

....

....

Evening Playbook

GRATITUDE:

List 3 things you are grateful for (which can include future manifestations):

1. ....
....

2. ....
....

3. ....
....

AFFIRMATIONS:

Write 3 affirmations:

1. ....
....

2. ....
....

3. ....
....

FEELINGS:

How did you feel today? ....

How do you feel now? ....

How do you intend to feel tomorrow? ....

INSPIRATION:

Did you receive inspiration today? ....

Describe what you were inspired to do or say ....
....

FOOD EXPERIMENT:

What single item of food did you experiment with today? ....

Describe how you felt? ....
....

Does your unique body process this food easily? ....

QUOTE OF THE DAY:

" If you've been reaching for a snack to soothe your negative emotions for your entire life, you can return to a balanced body within weeks. The momentum of a life-long habit can be reversed in just a few short weeks. This is due top the amazing restorative qualities of the body. Once you engage change, your cells respond by realigning themselves and balance is achieved. All it takes is a commitment to focus." *Joshua*

Morning Playbook

MEDITATION:

Duration ....   Type...

Time of Day ....   Satisfaction Level: 1   2   3   4   5   6   7   8   9   10

Notes: ....

....

APPRECIATION:

List 3 things you appreciate about your life:

1. ....

....

2. ....

....

3. ....

....

INTENTIONS:

Set your general intentions for the day:

....

....

....

....

....

....

Evening Playbook

GRATITUDE:

List 3 things you are grateful for (which can include future manifestations):

1. ....

....

2. ....

....

3. ....

....

AFFIRMATIONS:

Write 3 affirmations:

1. ....

....

2. ....

....

3. ....

....

FEELINGS:

How did you feel today? ....

How do you feel now? ....

How do you intend to feel tomorrow? ....

INSPIRATION:

Did you receive inspiration today? ....

Describe what you were inspired to do or say ....

....

FOOD EXPERIMENT:

What single item of food did you experiment with today?......................

Describe how you felt? ....

....

Does your unique body process this food easily? ....

QUOTE OF THE DAY:

66 When you are focused on something you want, the entire universe is there working with you. It might be difficult for you to comprehend, but that is how the system was designed. When you focus strongly on what is wanted, the universe stands with you and the power that created the universe is channeled through you." *Joshua*

Morning Playbook

MEDITATION:

Duration ....   Type...

Time of Day ....   Satisfaction Level: 1   2   3   4   5   6   7   8   9   10

Notes: ....

....

APPRECIATION:

List 3 things you appreciate about your life:

1. ....

   ....

2. ....

   ....

3. ....

   ....

INTENTIONS:

Set your general intentions for the day:

....

....

....

....

....

....

Evening Playbook

GRATITUDE:

List 3 things you are grateful for (which can include future manifestations):

1. ....
....

2. ....
....

3. ....
....

AFFIRMATIONS:

Write 3 affirmations:

1. ....
....

2. ....
....

3. ....
....

FEELINGS:

How did you feel today? ....

How do you feel now? ....

How do you intend to feel tomorrow? ....

INSPIRATION:

Did you receive inspiration today? ....

Describe what you were inspired to do or say ....
....

FOOD EXPERIMENT:

What single item of food did you experiment with today?.......................

Describe how you felt? ....
....

Does your unique body process this food easily? ....

QUOTE OF THE DAY:

" When you believe that it is all up to you alone to create anything you desire, whether that is a lean body, a loving relationship, a new house, a dream job or business, you set up a perspective that allows for the possibility of failure." *Joshua*

Morning Playbook

MEDITATION:

Duration .... Type...

Time of Day .... Satisfaction Level: 1 2 3 4 5 6 7 8 9 10

Notes: ....

....

APPRECIATION:

List 3 things you appreciate about your life:

1. ....

....

2. ....

....

3. ....

....

INTENTIONS:

Set your general intentions for the day:

....

....

....

....

....

....

Evening Playbook

GRATITUDE:

List 3 things you are grateful for (which can include future manifestations):

1. ....

   ....

2. ....

   ....

3. ....

   ....

AFFIRMATIONS:

Write 3 affirmations:

1. ....

   ....

2. ....

   ....

3. ....

   ....

FEELINGS:

How did you feel today? ....

How do you feel now? ....

How do you intend to feel tomorrow? ....

INSPIRATION:

Did you receive inspiration today? ....

Describe what you were inspired to do or say ....

....

FOOD EXPERIMENT:

What single item of food did you experiment with today?.....................

Describe how you felt? ....

....

Does your unique body process this food easily? ....

QUOTE OF THE DAY:

" If you believed you could not fail, you would engage the forces of the universe and together, you would be so powerful, so aligned, so confident, so effective that you could not fail. It would simply be out of the realm of possibility." *Joshua*

Morning Playbook

MEDITATION:

Duration ....   Type..

Time of Day ....   Satisfaction Level: 1 2 3 4 5 6 7 8 9 10

Notes: ....
....

APPRECIATION:

List 3 things you appreciate about your life:

1. ....
   ....
2. ....
   ....
3. ....
   ....

INTENTIONS:

Set your general intentions for the day:

....
....
....
....
....
....

Evening Playbook

GRATITUDE:

List 3 things you are grateful for (which can include future manifestations):

1. ....
....

2. ....
....

3. ....
....

AFFIRMATIONS:

Write 3 affirmations:

1. ....
....

2. ....
....

3. ....
....

FEELINGS:

How did you feel today? ....

How do you feel now? ....

How do you intend to feel tomorrow? ....

INSPIRATION:

Did you receive inspiration today? ....

Describe what you were inspired to do or say ....
....

FOOD EXPERIMENT:

What single item of food did you experiment with today? ....

Describe how you felt? ....
....

Does your unique body process this food easily? ....

QUOTE OF THE DAY:

❝ If you can get yourself to believe that you create your own reality, that you have a vast inner support network to back you, that the universe yields to your desires, that the power of focus aligns all your support behind you with one mission in mind, you can absolutely be, have, and do anything you desire in this reality. It is the basic design of the system." *Joshua*

Morning Playbook

MEDITATION:

Duration ....   Type..

Time of Day ....   Satisfaction Level: 1 2 3 4 5 6 7 8 9 10

Notes: ....
....

APPRECIATION:

List 3 things you appreciate about your life:

1. ....
....

2. ....
....

3. ....
....

INTENTIONS:

Set your general intentions for the day:

....
....
....
....
....
....

Evening Playbook

List 3 things you are grateful for (which can include future manifestations):

1. ....

   ....

2. ....

   ....

3. ....

   ....

AFFIRMATIONS:

Write 3 affirmations:

1. ....

   ....

2. ....

   ....

3. ....

   ....

FEELINGS:

How did you feel today? ....

How do you feel now? ....

How do you intend to feel tomorrow? ....

INSPIRATION:

Did you receive inspiration today? ....

Describe what you were inspired to do or say ....

....

FOOD EXPERIMENT:

What single item of food did you experiment with today? ....

Describe how you felt? ....

....

Does your unique body process this food easily? ....

QUOTE OF THE DAY:

" You are a unique expression of source. You are here to explore reality from a unique perspective. No other person has ever or will ever perceive reality as you are perceiving it right now. You are completely and absolutely unique to all the universe. Your unique experience of life adds to the sum total of the universe since each point of perspective is equally unique and all points of perspective are equally valid and valuable, one not more so than any other. Your complete and total uniqueness proves your worthiness and value to all that is." *Joshua*

Morning Playbook

MEDITATION:

Duration .... Type...

Time of Day .... Satisfaction Level: 1 2 3 4 5 6 7 8 9 10

Notes: ....

....

APPRECIATION:

List 3 things you appreciate about your life:

1. ....

   ....

2. ....

   ....

3. ....

   ....

INTENTIONS:

Set your general intentions for the day:

....

....

....

....

....

Evening Playbook

GRATITUDE:

List 3 things you are grateful for (which can include future manifestations):

1. ....
....

2. ....
....

3. ....
....

AFFIRMATIONS:

Write 3 affirmations:

1. ....
....

2. ....
....

3. ....
....

FEELINGS:

How did you feel today? ....

How do you feel now? ....

How do you intend to feel tomorrow? ....

INSPIRATION:

Did you receive inspiration today? ....

Describe what you were inspired to do or say ....
....

FOOD EXPERIMENT:

What single item of food did you experiment with today? ....

Describe how you felt? ....
....

Does your unique body process this food easily? ....

QUOTE OF THE DAY:

" You are worthy of all that you want. Your doubt that you are worthy is what causes much of your resistance. Fear and self-doubt are resistant in nature. Love, confidence, and ease are allowing in nature. When you experience self-doubt, you are feeling unworthy. When you experience confidence, you are feeling worthy. Worthy-feeling people allow what they want to flow to them. Unworthy-feeling people resist it because they fear receiving that which they are not worthy of." *Joshua*

Morning Playbook

MEDITATION:

Duration ....   Type..

Time of Day ....   Satisfaction Level: 1   2   3   4   5   6   7   8   9   10

Notes: ....

....

APPRECIATION:

List 3 things you appreciate about your life:

1. ....

   ....

2. ....

   ....

3. ....

   ....

INTENTIONS:

Set your general intentions for the day:

....

....

....

....

....

Evening Playbook

GRATITUDE:

List 3 things you are grateful for (which can include future manifestations):

1. ....
....

2. ....
....

3. ....
....

AFFIRMATIONS:

Write 3 affirmations:

1. ....
....

2. ....
....

3. ....
....

FEELINGS:

How did you feel today? ....

How do you feel now? ....

How do you intend to feel tomorrow? ....

INSPIRATION:

Did you receive inspiration today? ....

Describe what you were inspired to do or say ....
....

FOOD EXPERIMENT:

What single item of food did you experiment with today? ....

Describe how you felt? ....
....

Does your unique body process this food easily? ....

QUOTE OF THE DAY:

> "You are an eternal and limitless being of pure positive love. You are love. That's who you are. That's who everyone is. You are all part of source and source is pure love. Who you really are is a being of love. Who you are being right now, in your home, in your body, is something less than that. You are moving from who you are right now, to who you really are. You are an eternal and limitless being of pure positive love." *Joshua*

Morning Playbook

MEDITATION:

Duration ....   Type...

Time of Day ....   Satisfaction Level: 1 2 3 4 5 6 7 8 9 10

Notes: ....

....

APPRECIATION:

List 3 things you appreciate about your life:

1. ....

....

2. ....

....

3. ....

....

INTENTIONS:

Set your general intentions for the day:

....

....

....

....

....

....

Evening Playbook

GRATITUDE:

List 3 things you are grateful for (which can include future manifestations):

1. ....
....

2. ....
....

3. ....
....

AFFIRMATIONS:

Write 3 affirmations:

1. ....
....

2. ....
....

3. ....
....

FEELINGS:

How did you feel today? ....

How do you feel now? ....

How do you intend to feel tomorrow? ....

INSPIRATION:

Did you receive inspiration today? ....

Describe what you were inspired to do or say ....
....

FOOD EXPERIMENT:

What single item of food did you experiment with today?......................

Describe how you felt? ....
....

Does your unique body process this food easily? ....

QUOTE OF THE DAY:

"Your body is a representation of your thoughts, feelings, beliefs, and expectations, but it is not you. You can control certain functions of the body consciously, but the vast majority of its functions are done without your awareness. Your body is comprised of individual cells and each cell is an individual point of consciousness, just as alive as you are. Each cell seeks well-being just as you do. Each cell is here to live a joyful and expansive existence, just as you are." *Joshua*

Morning Playbook

MEDITATION:

Duration ....   Type...

Time of Day ....   Satisfaction Level: 1   2   3   4   5   6   7   8   9   10

Notes: ....

....

APPRECIATION:

List 3 things you appreciate about your life:

1. ....

   ....

2. ....

   ....

3. ....

   ....

INTENTIONS:

Set your general intentions for the day:

....

....

....

....

....

....

Evening Playbook

GRATITUDE:

List 3 things you are grateful for (which can include future manifestations):

1. ....

   ....

2. ....

   ....

3. ....

   ....

AFFIRMATIONS:

Write 3 affirmations:

1. ....

   ....

2. ....

   ....

3. ....

   ....

FEELINGS:

How did you feel today? ....

How do you feel now? ....

How do you intend to feel tomorrow? ....

INSPIRATION:

Did you receive inspiration today? ....

Describe what you were inspired to do or say ....

....

FOOD EXPERIMENT:

What single item of food did you experiment with today?.....................

Describe how you felt? ....

....

Does your unique body process this food easily? ....

QUOTE OF THE DAY:

" If you knew your worth, you would not make choices that did not fully align with who you know yourself to be. If you knew you were the creator of your own reality, you would not say things that did not align with who you are. If you understood your power, you would not settle for something less than the highest and most elegant manifestation of what you wanted. If you understood your perfection (and the whole idea of perfection), you would not discount any aspect of yourself and you would never compare yourself to anyone else." *Joshua*

Morning Playbook

MEDITATION:

Duration ....   Type...

Time of Day ....   Satisfaction Level: 1   2   3   4   5   6   7   8   9   10

Notes: ....

....

APPRECIATION:

List 3 things you appreciate about your life:

1. ....

....

2. ....

....

3. ....

....

INTENTIONS:

Set your general intentions for the day:

....

....

....

....

....

Evening Playbook

GRATITUDE:

List 3 things you are grateful for (which can include future manifestations):

1. ....
....

2. ....
....

3. ....
....

AFFIRMATIONS:

Write 3 affirmations:

1. ....
....

2. ....
....

3. ....
....

FEELINGS:

How did you feel today? ....

How do you feel now? ....

How do you intend to feel tomorrow? ....

INSPIRATION:

Did you receive inspiration today? ....

Describe what you were inspired to do or say ....
....

FOOD EXPERIMENT:

What single item of food did you experiment with today?................................

Describe how you felt? ....
....

Does your unique body process this food easily? ....

QUOTE OF THE DAY:

❝ You do not want a lean body. What you want is to feel good. You do not want money, love, a career, or things. What you really want is to feel good. This is a feeling reality. All you are ever doing is either feeling good or not so good. Nothing is more important than how you feel. If you felt good right now, wouldn't that be nice? If you felt wonderful right now, what would be better than that? When you want something, it's not the thing you want, it's the feeling you think that thing will bring." *Joshua*

Morning Playbook

MEDITATION:

Duration .... Type...

Time of Day .... Satisfaction Level: 1 2 3 4 5 6 7 8 9 10

Notes: ....

....

APPRECIATION:

List 3 things you appreciate about your life:

1. ....

....

2. ....

....

3. ....

....

INTENTIONS:

Set your general intentions for the day:

....

....

....

....

....

Evening Playbook

GRATITUDE:

List 3 things you are grateful for (which can include future manifestations):

1. ....

   ....

2. ....

   ....

3. ....

   ....

AFFIRMATIONS:

Write 3 affirmations:

1. ....

   ....

2. ....

   ....

3. ....

   ....

FEELINGS:

How did you feel today? ....

How do you feel now? ....

How do you intend to feel tomorrow? ....

INSPIRATION:

Did you receive inspiration today? ....

Describe what you were inspired to do or say ....

....

FOOD EXPERIMENT:

What single item of food did you experiment with today?....................................

Describe how you felt? ....

....

Does your unique body process this food easily? ....

QUOTE OF THE DAY:

❝ This is an attractive universe, not a resistant one. You attract what you want (or don't want) by your focus of attention. If you don't like your body as it is now, you tend to think about, complain about, and be ashamed about the things you don't like. As you place your focus on these things, the universe via the Law of Attraction brings more of what you don't like." *Joshua*

Morning Playbook

MEDITATION:

Duration ....   Type...

Time of Day ....   Satisfaction Level: 1   2   3   4   5   6   7   8   9   10

Notes: ....

....

APPRECIATION:

List 3 things you appreciate about your life:

1. ....

    ....

2. ....

    ....

3. ....

    ....

INTENTIONS:

Set your general intentions for the day:

....

....

....

....

....

....

Evening Playbook

List 3 things you are grateful for (which can include future manifestations):

1. ....
....
2. ....
....
3. ....
....

AFFIRMATIONS:

Write 3 affirmations:

1. ....
....
2. ....
....
3. ....
....

FEELINGS:

How did you feel today? ....

How do you feel now? ....

How do you intend to feel tomorrow? ....

INSPIRATION:

Did you receive inspiration today? ....

Describe what you were inspired to do or say ....

....

FOOD EXPERIMENT:

What single item of food did you experiment with today?................................

Describe how you felt? ....

....

Does your unique body process this food easily? ....

QUOTE OF THE DAY:

" The only way to get anything you want is to allow it to come. The only way to allow anything to come is by creating an environment where it's easy to allow. Are you allowing when you are hating the fat? No, you are resisting. Are you allowing when you are ashamed of your body? No. you are resisting. Are you allowing when you are starving yourself? No, you are resisting." *Joshua*

Morning Playbook

MEDITATION:

Duration ....   Type...

Time of Day ....   Satisfaction Level: 1   2   3   4   5   6   7   8   9   10

Notes: ....

....

APPRECIATION:

List 3 things you appreciate about your life:

1. ....

   ....

2. ....

   ....

3. ....

   ....

INTENTIONS:

Set your general intentions for the day:

....

....

....

....

....

....

Evening Playbook

GRATITUDE:

List 3 things you are grateful for (which can include future manifestations):

1. ....

   ....

2. ....

   ....

3. ....

   ....

AFFIRMATIONS:

Write 3 affirmations:

1. ....

   ....

2. ....

   ....

3. ....

   ....

FEELINGS:

How did you feel today?...

How do you feel now?..

How do you intend to feel tomorrow? ....

INSPIRATION:

Did you receive inspiration today? ....

Describe what you were inspired to do or say ....

....

FOOD EXPERIMENT:

What single item of food did you experiment with today?..............................

Describe how you felt? ....

....

Does your unique body process this food easily? ....

QUOTE OF THE DAY:

" It's not the events that cause you to feel bad; it's your perspective. The things that bring up negative emotion for you are not bad things in and of themselves. They are just the way they are. They are neutral. It's you who decides if something is good or bad, right or wrong." *Joshua*

Morning Playbook

MEDITATION:

Duration .... Type..

Time of Day .... Satisfaction Level: 1 2 3 4 5 6 7 8 9 10

Notes: ....

....

APPRECIATION:

List 3 things you appreciate about your life:

1. ....

   ....

2. ....

   ....

3. ....

   ....

INTENTIONS:

Set your general intentions for the day:

....

....

....

....

....

....

Evening Playbook

GRATITUDE:

List 3 things you are grateful for (which can include future manifestations):

1. ....
....
2. ....
....
3. ....
....

AFFIRMATIONS:

Write 3 affirmations:

1. ....
....
2. ....
....
3. ....
....

FEELINGS:

How did you feel today? ....

How do you feel now? ....

How do you intend to feel tomorrow? ....

INSPIRATION:

Did you receive inspiration today? ....

Describe what you were inspired to do or say ....
....

FOOD EXPERIMENT:

What single item of food did you experiment with today?.................

Describe how you felt? ....
....

Does your unique body process this food easily? ....

QUOTE OF THE DAY:

" Your perspective is your story. You can tell a story that aligns with who you really are and what you really want or you can make up a story that conflicts with what you want. It's up to you. You can choose a perspective that's empowering or limited. It's your choice. You can choose to be engaged in the world around you or frozen with fear. It's your choice. Lean in and move through the fear and your self-imposed limitations will fade away." *Joshua*

Morning Playbook

MEDITATION:

Duration ....   Type..

Time of Day ....   Satisfaction Level: 1   2   3   4   5   6   7   8   9   10

Notes: ....

....

APPRECIATION:

List 3 things you appreciate about your life:

1. ....

   ....

2. ....

   ....

3. ....

   ....

INTENTIONS:

Set your general intentions for the day:

....

....

....

....

....

....

Evening Playbook

GRATITUDE:

List 3 things you are grateful for (which can include future manifestations):

1. ....

....

2. ....

....

3. ....

....

AFFIRMATIONS:

Write 3 affirmations:

1. ....

....

2. ....

....

3. ....

....

FEELINGS:

How did you feel today? ....

How do you feel now? ....

How do you intend to feel tomorrow? ....

INSPIRATION:

Did you receive inspiration today? ....

Describe what you were inspired to do or say ....

....

FOOD EXPERIMENT:

What single item of food did you experiment with today? ....

Describe how you felt? ....

....

Does your unique body process this food easily? ....

QUOTE OF THE DAY:

" Negative emotion need not be painful when you see it as a message rather than a punishment. It's no longer painful when you can analyze it and release it rather than hang onto it. Negative emotion is no longer limiting when you can dismiss it quickly by choosing the proper perspective. When negative emotion no longer reigns over your life, your life expands dramatically." *Joshua*

Morning Playbook

MEDITATION:

Duration .... Type...

Time of Day .... Satisfaction Level: 1 2 3 4 5 6 7 8 9 10

Notes: ....

....

APPRECIATION:

List 3 things you appreciate about your life:

1. ....

....

2. ....

....

3. ....

....

INTENTIONS:

Set your general intentions for the day:

....

....

....

....

....

....

Evening Playbook

GRATITUDE:

List 3 things you are grateful for (which can include future manifestations):

1. ....

....

2. ....

....

3. ....

....

AFFIRMATIONS:

Write 3 affirmations:

1. ....

....

2. ....

....

3. ....

....

FEELINGS:

How did you feel today? ....

How do you feel now? ....

How do you intend to feel tomorrow? ....

INSPIRATION:

Did you receive inspiration today? ....

Describe what you were inspired to do or say ....

....

FOOD EXPERIMENT:

What single item of food did you experiment with today?................................

Describe how you felt? ....

....

Does your unique body process this food easily? ....

QUOTE OF THE DAY:

" Can you imagine accepting negative emotion as a gift? It seems impossible, doesn't it? How can you become so aware of yourself, of the world around you, and of your own fears and insecurities that you actually feel good when you receive negative emotion? It's all in your expectations, your attitude, and your approach to life." *Joshua*

Morning Playbook

MEDITATION:

Duration .... Type...

Time of Day .... Satisfaction Level: 1 2 3 4 5 6 7 8 9 10

Notes: ....

....

APPRECIATION:

List 3 things you appreciate about your life:

1. ....

   ....

2. ....

   ....

3. ....

   ....

INTENTIONS:

Set your general intentions for the day:

....

....

....

....

....

....

....

Evening Playbook

GRATITUDE:

List 3 things you are grateful for (which can include future manifestations):

1. ....
....
2. ....
....
3. ....
....

AFFIRMATIONS:

Write 3 affirmations:

1. ....
....
2. ....
....
3. ....
....

FEELINGS:

How did you feel today? ....

How do you feel now? ....

How do you intend to feel tomorrow? ....

INSPIRATION:

Did you receive inspiration today? ....

Describe what you were inspired to do or say ....
....

FOOD EXPERIMENT:

What single item of food did you experiment with today?............................

Describe how you felt? ....
....

Does your unique body process this food easily? ....

QUOTE OF THE DAY:

66 Even the tiniest vibration of something you consider mildly bad or wrong affects your vibration. Imagine cooking a soup. You stir in all the ingredients and let it simmer. Soon they come together to create a wonderful flavor. Now you see a bottle of vinegar, which you do not like, but for some reason you decide to add it to your soup. Not much, just a few drops. How does the soup taste now? It's a different flavor, isn't it? It's not a bad flavor, it's just one you do not like. We are not saying it's bad or wrong to pay attention to things you do not prefer; we are only saying that you're adding something to the mix that is out of alignment with what you want. You're cooking a different soup." *Joshua*

Morning Playbook

MEDITATION:

Duration .... Type..

Time of Day .... Satisfaction Level: 1 2 3 4 5 6 7 8 9 10

Notes: ....
....

APPRECIATION:

List 3 things you appreciate about your life:

1. ....
   ....

2. ....
   ....

3. ....
   ....

INTENTIONS:

Set your general intentions for the day:

....
....
....
....
....

Evening Playbook

GRATITUDE:

List 3 things you are grateful for (which can include future manifestations):

1. ....
....

2. ....
....

3. ....
....

AFFIRMATIONS:

Write 3 affirmations:

1. ....
....

2. ....
....

3. ....
....

FEELINGS:

How did you feel today? ....

How do you feel now? ....

How do you intend to feel tomorrow? ....

INSPIRATION:

Did you receive inspiration today? ....

Describe what you were inspired to do or say ....
....

FOOD EXPERIMENT:

What single item of food did you experiment with today? ....

Describe how you felt? ....
....

Does your unique body process this food easily? ....

QUOTE OF THE DAY:

" In order to slow the momentum of the unwanted, it is important to refrain from speaking about the things you think are bad, wrong, or broken. Remove your attention from them. Stop believing they are bad or wrong. Start seeing some positive aspects of these things. Change your perspective on the subject. Disengage with those who want to talk about things they believe are wrong. Change the conversation or leave the room." *Joshua*

Morning Playbook

MEDITATION:

Duration ....   Type...

Time of Day ....   Satisfaction Level: 1   2   3   4   5   6   7   8   9   10

Notes: ....

....

APPRECIATION:

List 3 things you appreciate about your life:

1. ....

   ....

2. ....

   ....

3. ....

   ....

INTENTIONS:

Set your general intentions for the day:

....

....

....

....

....

....

Evening Playbook

GRATITUDE:

List 3 things you are grateful for (which can include future manifestations):

1. ....
....

2. ....
....

3. ....
....

AFFIRMATIONS:

Write 3 affirmations:

1. ....
....

2. ....
....

3. ....
....

FEELINGS:

How did you feel today? ....

How do you feel now? ....

How do you intend to feel tomorrow? ....

INSPIRATION:

Did you receive inspiration today? ....

Describe what you were inspired to do or say ....
....

FOOD EXPERIMENT:

What single item of food did you experiment with today?.............................

Describe how you felt? ....
....

Does your unique body process this food easily? ....

QUOTE OF THE DAY:

" Your words are powerful. Use them with thought and intention. Intend to discuss topics of interest and inspiration. Intend to speak eloquently about things you like. Intend to remove yourself from any subject that is not appealing to you. Intend to remove your attention from unwanted things, even if you're a little curious. Realize that you do not need to be informed about anything that is not vibrationally uplifting. Focus on whatever you think is positive and remove your attention from whatever you personally view as negative." *Joshua*

Morning Playbook

MEDITATION:

Duration ....   Type...

Time of Day ....   Satisfaction Level: 1   2   3   4   5   6   7   8   9   10

Notes: ....

....

APPRECIATION:

List 3 things you appreciate about your life:

1. ....

   ....

2. ....

   ....

3. ....

   ....

INTENTIONS:

Set your general intentions for the day:

....

....

....

....

....

Evening Playbook

GRATITUDE:

List 3 things you are grateful for (which can include future manifestations):

1. ....

....

2. ....

....

3. ....

....

AFFIRMATIONS:

Write 3 affirmations:

1. ....

....

2. ....

....

3. ....

....

FEELINGS:

How did you feel today? ....

How do you feel now? ....

How do you intend to feel tomorrow? ....

INSPIRATION:

Did you receive inspiration today? ....

Describe what you were inspired to do or say ....

....

FOOD EXPERIMENT:

What single item of food did you experiment with today?........................

Describe how you felt? ....

....

Does your unique body process this food easily? ....

QUOTE OF THE DAY:

" As you transition from a victim mentality to a creator mentality, you are really moving from irresponsibility to full responsibility. In the old approach, other things outside yourself had a lot to do with what happened. In this new approach, you are responsible for everything that happens in your world. You are now the center of your universe. You now control every single little thing that presents itself in your reality." *Joshua*

Morning Playbook

MEDITATION:

Duration .... Type...

Time of Day .... Satisfaction Level: 1 2 3 4 5 6 7 8 9 10

Notes: ....

....

APPRECIATION:

List 3 things you appreciate about your life:

1. ....

....

2. ....

....

3. ....

....

INTENTIONS:

Set your general intentions for the day:

....

....

....

....

....

....

Evening Playbook

GRATITUDE:

List 3 things you are grateful for (which can include future manifestations):

1. ....

    ....

2. ....

    ....

3. ....

    ....

AFFIRMATIONS:

Write 3 affirmations:

1. ....

    ....

2. ....

    ....

3. ....

    ....

FEELINGS:

How did you feel today? ....

How do you feel now? ....

How do you intend to feel tomorrow? ....

INSPIRATION:

Did you receive inspiration today? ....

Describe what you were inspired to do or say ....

....

FOOD EXPERIMENT:

What single item of food did you experiment with today?......................

Describe how you felt? ....

....

Does your unique body process this food easily? ....

QUOTE OF THE DAY:

" You can easily spot the people who naturally abide by the laws of the universe. They are happy, positive, easygoing, and seem to go with the flow of life. They are optimists. They are confident. They love themselves and others. They see the good and do not spend much time on things they do not like. You might call them Pollyanna, yet this is the approach to life that naturally aligns with the forces of the universe." *Joshua*

Morning Playbook

MEDITATION:

Duration ....   Type...

Time of Day ....   Satisfaction Level: 1   2   3   4   5   6   7   8   9   10

Notes: ....

....

APPRECIATION:

List 3 things you appreciate about your life:

1. ....

   ....

2. ....

   ....

3. ....

   ....

INTENTIONS:

Set your general intentions for the day:

....

....

....

....

....

....

Evening Playbook

GRATITUDE:

List 3 things you are grateful for (which can include future manifestations):

1. ....

....

2. ....

....

3. ....

....

AFFIRMATIONS:

Write 3 affirmations:

1. ....

....

2. ....

....

3. ....

....

FEELINGS:

How did you feel today? ....

How do you feel now? ....

How do you intend to feel tomorrow? ....

INSPIRATION:

Did you receive inspiration today? ....

Describe what you were inspired to do or say ....

....

FOOD EXPERIMENT:

What single item of food did you experiment with today?................................

Describe how you felt? ....

....

Does your unique body process this food easily? ....

QUOTE OF THE DAY:

> " There is a flow to life. The universe is constantly moving you in the direction toward what is wanted. You have a very limited point of view. From your perspective, you cannot see very far down the road. You cannot know what is being set up. You do not know how your beliefs must be changed. However, the universe knows it all. If you are to go with the flow of life, you must come to understand that everything is happening for you and nothing is happening to you." *Joshua*

Morning Playbook

MEDITATION:

Duration ....   Type..

Time of Day ....   Satisfaction Level: 1   2   3   4   5   6   7   8   9   10

Notes: ....

....

APPRECIATION:

List 3 things you appreciate about your life:

1. ....

   ....

2. ....

   ....

3. ....

   ....

INTENTIONS:

Set your general intentions for the day:

....

....

....

....

....

....

Evening Playbook

GRATITUDE:

List 3 things you are grateful for (which can include future manifestations):

1. ....

....

2. ....

....

3. ....

....

AFFIRMATIONS:

Write 3 affirmations:

1. ....

....

2. ....

....

3. ....

....

FEELINGS:

How did you feel today? ....

How do you feel now? ....

How do you intend to feel tomorrow? ....

INSPIRATION:

Did you receive inspiration today? ....

Describe what you were inspired to do or say ....

....

FOOD EXPERIMENT:

What single item of food did you experiment with today?...................

Describe how you felt? ....

....

Does your unique body process this food easily? ....

QUOTE OF THE DAY:

" Give up your idea of effort and struggle. If it is difficult, if it is painful, if it is a struggle, then you are not engaging the forces of the universe and you're not going with the flow of life. If you are doing something you do not enjoy in the hope you will lose weight, you cannot create a lean body that will remain lean for very long." *Joshua*

Morning Playbook

MEDITATION:

Duration .... Type..

Time of Day .... Satisfaction Level: 1 2 3 4 5 6 7 8 9 10

Notes: ....
....

APPRECIATION:

List 3 things you appreciate about your life:

1. ....
....

2. ....
....

3. ....
....

INTENTIONS:

Set your general intentions for the day:

....
....
....
....
....
....

Evening Playbook

GRATITUDE:
List 3 things you are grateful for (which can include future manifestations):

1. ....
....

2. ....
....

3. ....
....

AFFIRMATIONS:
Write 3 affirmations:

1. ....
....

2. ....
....

3. ....
....

FEELINGS:
How did you feel today? ....

How do you feel now? ....

How do you intend to feel tomorrow? ....

INSPIRATION:
Did you receive inspiration today? ....

Describe what you were inspired to do or say ....
....

FOOD EXPERIMENT:
What single item of food did you experiment with today?............................

Describe how you felt? ....
....

Does your unique body process this food easily? ....

QUOTE OF THE DAY:

> When you hate your body as it is, you are placing a lot of attention on what is and the universe responds to that attention. There is no good or bad in the universe; everything is neutral. The universe seeks to bring you that which you are paying attention to. It assumes that if you are focused on something, you must like that thing, otherwise you would focus your attention elsewhere. Doesn't that make sense? When you focus your attention on something you think is wrong, the universe brings more of that into your life." *Joshua*

Morning Playbook

MEDITATION:

Duration ....   Type...

Time of Day ....   Satisfaction Level: 1 2 3 4 5 6 7 8 9 10

Notes: ....

....

APPRECIATION:

List 3 things you appreciate about your life:

1. ....

....

2. ....

....

3. ....

....

INTENTIONS:

Set your general intentions for the day:

....

....

....

....

....

Evening Playbook

GRATITUDE:

List 3 things you are grateful for (which can include future manifestations):

1. ....
....
2. ....
....
3. ....
....

AFFIRMATIONS:

Write 3 affirmations:

1. ....
....
2. ....
....
3. ....
....

FEELINGS:

How did you feel today? ....

How do you feel now? ....

How do you intend to feel tomorrow? ....

INSPIRATION:

Did you receive inspiration today? ....

Describe what you were inspired to do or say ....
....

FOOD EXPERIMENT:

What single item of food did you experiment with today? ....

Describe how you felt? ....
....

Does your unique body process this food easily? ....

QUOTE OF THE DAY:

" The reason nothing has changed for you is because you haven't changed. Until you make some fundamental changes, your outer reality will not change. Nothing will change. However, once you make some small changes to who you are being right now, then everything changes. Not only will your body improve, but everything else will improve right along with it. Your relationships will improve, your finances will improve, your mood will improve, your health will improve. Everything gets better when you decide to become who you really are." *Joshua*

Morning Playbook

MEDITATION:

Duration .... Type..

Time of Day .... Satisfaction Level: 1   2   3   4   5   6   7   8   9   10

Notes: ....

....

APPRECIATION:

List 3 things you appreciate about your life:

1. ....

   ....

2. ....

   ....

3. ....

   ....

INTENTIONS:

Set your general intentions for the day:

....

....

....

....

....

Evening Playbook

GRATITUDE:

List 3 things you are grateful for (which can include future manifestations):

1. ....
....
2. ....
....
3. ....
....

AFFIRMATIONS:

Write 3 affirmations:

1. ....
....
2. ....
....
3. ....
....

FEELINGS:

How did you feel today? ....

How do you feel now? ....

How do you intend to feel tomorrow? ....

INSPIRATION:

Did you receive inspiration today? ....

Describe what you were inspired to do or say ....
....

FOOD EXPERIMENT:

What single item of food did you experiment with today? ....

Describe how you felt? ....
....

Does your unique body process this food easily? ....

QUOTE OF THE DAY:

> " Your outer reality is a representation of how you feel on the inside. If you feel bad on the inside, your conditions, no matter how they look, will continue to cause you to feel bad. They are simply and only a reflection of how you feel on the inside. That's it. You could make an effort and physically change the appearance of your outer conditions and for a while you might feel better. But the conditions are not creating a change within you; you are creating the change in your outside conditions and therefore no real inner change is taking place. Soon enough, when the illusion of change goes away, things will start to feel the way they always did and everything in your outer reality will feel a lot like it always did." *Joshua*

Morning Playbook

MEDITATION:

Duration ....   Type..

Time of Day ....   Satisfaction Level: 1   2   3   4   5   6   7   8   9   10

Notes: ....

....

APPRECIATION:

List 3 things you appreciate about your life:

1. ....

   ....

2. ....

   ....

3. ....

   ....

INTENTIONS:

Set your general intentions for the day:

....

....

....

....

Evening Playbook

GRATITUDE:

List 3 things you are grateful for (which can include future manifestations):

1. ....
....
2. ....
....
3. ....
....

AFFIRMATIONS:

Write 3 affirmations:

1. ....
....
2. ....
....
3. ....
....

FEELINGS:

How did you feel today? ....

How do you feel now? ....

How do you intend to feel tomorrow? ....

INSPIRATION:

Did you receive inspiration today? ....

Describe what you were inspired to do or say ....
....

FOOD EXPERIMENT:

What single item of food did you experiment with today?.........................

Describe how you felt? ....
....

Does your unique body process this food easily? ....

QUOTE OF THE DAY:

"Change is not as difficult as it appears. You are constantly in a state of change. You are a fluid being, always and forever changing. You could not possibly be static for even a moment in time because with each new moment, you are forever changed. Every cell in your body is changing also. Millions of cells are dying and new ones are replacing them. Your body is in a constant state of flux. It is a completely new body every moment as it loses and receives cells. You cannot keep yourself from changing, so why not embrace change?" *Joshua*

Morning Playbook

MEDITATION:

Duration .... Type ....

Time of Day .... Satisfaction Level: 1 2 3 4 5 6 7 8 9 10

Notes: ....

....

APPRECIATION:

List 3 things you appreciate about your life:

1. ....

....

2. ....

....

3. ....

....

INTENTIONS:

Set your general intentions for the day:

....

....

....

....

....

Evening Playbook

GRATITUDE:

List 3 things you are grateful for (which can include future manifestations):

1. ....
   ....
2. ....
   ....
3. ....
   ....

AFFIRMATIONS:

Write 3 affirmations:

1. ....
   ....
2. ....
   ....
3. ....
   ....

FEELINGS:

How did you feel today? ....

How do you feel now? ....

How do you intend to feel tomorrow? ....

INSPIRATION:

Did you receive inspiration today? ....

Describe what you were inspired to do or say ....
....

FOOD EXPERIMENT:

What single item of food did you experiment with today? ....

Describe how you felt? ....
....

Does your unique body process this food easily? ....

QUOTE OF THE DAY:

66 Typical diets all seek to change the outer conditions. If the inner feelings are not substantially changed, the outer conditions will always go back to how they were or even get worse. Long-term change must come from the inside. It is your feelings that create your reality." *Joshua*

Morning Playbook

MEDITATION:

Duration .... Type ....

Time of Day .... Satisfaction Level: 1   2   3   4   5   6   7   8   9   10

Notes: ....
....

APPRECIATION:

List 3 things you appreciate about your life:

1. ....
....

2. ....
....

3. ....
....

INTENTIONS:

Set your general intentions for the day:

....
....
....
....
....
....

Evening Playbook

GRATITUDE:
List 3 things you are grateful for (which can include future manifestations):

1. ....
....

2. ....
....

3. ....
....

AFFIRMATIONS:
Write 3 affirmations:

1. ....
....

2. ....
....

3. ....
....

FEELINGS:
How did you feel today? ....

How do you feel now? ....

How do you intend to feel tomorrow? ....

INSPIRATION:
Did you receive inspiration today? ....

Describe what you were inspired to do or say ....
....

FOOD EXPERIMENT:
What single item of food did you experiment with today?...............

Describe how you felt? ....
....

Does your unique body process this food easily? ....

QUOTE OF THE DAY:

" Fear is what keeps you from expressing who you really are. You want to fit in. You want to be accepted. You want to be loved. So you try to diminish the outstanding and unique qualities of yourself in fear of standing out and being different. Let's face it together. You are different. You are unique. You do have special gifts and talents and a unique personality. You have a truly unique outlook on life. You have a perspective that has never existed in the history of the world and will never exist again. You are special, unique, worthy, and important. Your life adds to the expansion of the universe. Without you, the universe would be less than it is now." *Joshua*

Morning Playbook

MEDITATION:

Duration .... Type..

Time of Day .... Satisfaction Level: 1 2 3 4 5 6 7 8 9 10

Notes: ....

....

APPRECIATION:

List 3 things you appreciate about your life:

1. ....

....

2. ....

....

3. ....

....

INTENTIONS:

Set your general intentions for the day:

....

....

....

....

Evening Playbook

GRATITUDE:

List 3 things you are grateful for (which can include future manifestations):

1. ....
....

2. ....
....

3. ....
....

AFFIRMATIONS:

Write 3 affirmations:

1. ....
....

2. ....
....

3. ....
....

FEELINGS:

How did you feel today? ....

How do you feel now? ....

How do you intend to feel tomorrow? ....

INSPIRATION:

Did you receive inspiration today? ....

Describe what you were inspired to do or say ....
....

FOOD EXPERIMENT:

What single item of food did you experiment with today? ....

Describe how you felt? ....
....

Does your unique body process this food easily? ....

QUOTE OF THE DAY:

"Very strong desire will overcome strong and entrenched limiting beliefs. If you have ever heard a story of a mother who lifted a car off her child, this is an example of a very strong desire overcoming very strong limiting beliefs. Any desire will be manifested by the universe as long as it is stronger than the limiting beliefs. You can have, be, and do anything you want in this reality as long as your desire is more robust than your limiting beliefs. Increase the power of your desires while simultaneously reducing the intensity of your limiting beliefs." *Joshua*

Morning Playbook

MEDITATION:

Duration .... Type...

Time of Day .... Satisfaction Level: 1 2 3 4 5 6 7 8 9 10

Notes: ....
....

APPRECIATION:

List 3 things you appreciate about your life:

1. ....
....

2. ....
....

3. ....
....

INTENTIONS:

Set your general intentions for the day:

....
....
....
....
....

Evening Playbook

GRATITUDE:

List 3 things you are grateful for (which can include future manifestations):

1. ....
....
2. ....
....
3. ....
....

AFFIRMATIONS:

Write 3 affirmations:

1. ....
....
2. ....
....
3. ....
....

FEELINGS:

How did you feel today? ....

How do you feel now? ....

How do you intend to feel tomorrow? ....

INSPIRATION:

Did you receive inspiration today? ....

Describe what you were inspired to do or say ....
....

FOOD EXPERIMENT:

What single item of food did you experiment with today? ....

Describe how you felt? ....
....

Does your unique body process this food easily? ....

QUOTE OF THE DAY:

66 Your desire is really up to you. The universe will help you reduce your limiting beliefs by placing you in situations where you have the opportunity to confront them and, through analysis, reduce their intensity. Reduce the intensity of your limiting beliefs and you automatically increase the chances that your desire will manifest." *Joshua*

Morning Playbook

MEDITATION:

Duration .... Type...

Time of Day .... Satisfaction Level: 1 2 3 4 5 6 7 8 9 10

Notes: ....

....

APPRECIATION:

List 3 things you appreciate about your life:

1. ....

....

2. ....

....

3. ....

....

INTENTIONS:

Set your general intentions for the day:

....

....

....

....

....

....

Evening Playbook

GRATITUDE:

List 3 things you are grateful for (which can include future manifestations):

1. ....

   ....

2. ....

   ....

3. ....

   ....

AFFIRMATIONS:

Write 3 affirmations:

1. ....

   ....

2. ....

   ....

3. ....

   ....

FEELINGS:

How did you feel today? ....

How do you feel now? ....

How do you intend to feel tomorrow? ....

INSPIRATION:

Did you receive inspiration today? ....

Describe what you were inspired to do or say ....

....

FOOD EXPERIMENT:

What single item of food did you experiment with today?.....................................

Describe how you felt? ....

....

Does your unique body process this food easily? ....

QUOTE OF THE DAY:

❝ If you knew that nothing ever happens to you, but that it always happens for you, you could learn to analyze every condition. With this perspective in mind, you would regain access to love-based channels and you could make decisions based in love. You would have access to empowering thoughts and your actions would be inspired from a place of feeling good. You would stop sabotaging yourself and you would engage the leverage of universal powers. You would be unstoppable." *Joshua*

Morning Playbook

MEDITATION:

Duration .... Type..

Time of Day .... Satisfaction Level: 1 2 3 4 5 6 7 8 9 10

Notes: ....

....

APPRECIATION:

List 3 things you appreciate about your life:

1. ....

   ....

2. ....

   ....

3. ....

   ....

INTENTIONS:

Set your general intentions for the day:

....

....

....

....

....

Evening Playbook

GRATITUDE:

List 3 things you are grateful for (which can include future manifestations):

1. ....
....

2. ....
....

3. ....
....

AFFIRMATIONS:

Write 3 affirmations:

1. ....
....

2. ....
....

3. ....
....

FEELINGS:

How did you feel today? ....

How do you feel now? ....

How do you intend to feel tomorrow? ....

INSPIRATION:

Did you receive inspiration today? ....

Describe what you were inspired to do or say ....
....

FOOD EXPERIMENT:

What single item of food did you experiment with today?.................

Describe how you felt? ....
....

Does your unique body process this food easily? ....

QUOTE OF THE DAY:

" There are two spectrums of thought available to you at any moment in time. If you feel good, you have access to a wide range of love-based thoughts and ideas depending on how good you feel. When you are fully engaged in your passion, be it art, music, business, conversation, research, etc., you have access to the very top of the spectrum. In these times of bliss, you are a vibrational match to high-vibrational thoughts and ideas." *Joshua*

Morning Playbook

MEDITATION:

Duration .... Type...

Time of Day .... Satisfaction Level: 1 2 3 4 5 6 7 8 9 10

Notes: ....

....

APPRECIATION:

List 3 things you appreciate about your life:

1. ....

   ....

2. ....

   ....

3. ....

   ....

INTENTIONS:

Set your general intentions for the day:

....

....

....

....

....

....

Evening Playbook

GRATITUDE:

List 3 things you are grateful for (which can include future manifestations):

1. ....
....

2. ....
....

3. ....
....

AFFIRMATIONS:

Write 3 affirmations:

1. ....
....

2. ....
....

3. ....
....

FEELINGS:

How did you feel today? ....

How do you feel now? ....

How do you intend to feel tomorrow? ....

INSPIRATION:

Did you receive inspiration today? ....

Describe what you were inspired to do or say ....
....

FOOD EXPERIMENT:

What single item of food did you experiment with today?...............

Describe how you felt? ....
....

Does your unique body process this food easily? ....

QUOTE OF THE DAY:

" If you found yourself in a state of fear and you could stop and analyze the situation and see that the fear is false because it is irrational, then you could choose a higher perspective and reach for love-based thoughts. These thoughts would then lead you to other love-based thoughts, words, and inspired action." *Joshua*

Morning Playbook

MEDITATION:

Duration .... Type...

Time of Day .... Satisfaction Level: 1 2 3 4 5 6 7 8 9 10

Notes: ....

....

APPRECIATION:

List 3 things you appreciate about your life:

1. ....

....

2. ....

....

3. ....

....

INTENTIONS:

Set your general intentions for the day:

....

....

....

....

....

....

Evening Playbook

GRATITUDE:

List 3 things you are grateful for (which can include future manifestations):

1. ....

....

2. ....

....

3. ....

....

AFFIRMATIONS:

Write 3 affirmations:

1. ....

....

2. ....

....

3. ....

....

FEELINGS:

How did you feel today? ....

How do you feel now? ....

How do you intend to feel tomorrow? ....

INSPIRATION:

Did you receive inspiration today? ....

Describe what you were inspired to do or say ....

....

FOOD EXPERIMENT:

What single item of food did you experiment with today?..............................

Describe how you felt? ....

....

Does your unique body process this food easily? ....

QUOTE OF THE DAY:

" Changing your state of being is an inner change. Change made from the inside affects the outside conditions. You have the knowledge and the tools you need to make significant inner changes that then utilize the forces of the universe to create the life experience you truly desire. It is all a mater of perspective and this is an approach to life that is in full alignment of universal laws." *Joshua*

Morning Playbook

MEDITATION:

Duration .... Type...

Time of Day .... Satisfaction Level: 1 2 3 4 5 6 7 8 9 10

Notes: ....
....

APPRECIATION:

List 3 things you appreciate about your life:

1. ....
   ....

2. ....
   ....

3. ....
   ....

INTENTIONS:

Set your general intentions for the day:

....
....
....
....
....
....

Evening Playbook

GRATITUDE:

List 3 things you are grateful for (which can include future manifestations):

1. ....
....

2. ....
....

3. ....
....

AFFIRMATIONS:

Write 3 affirmations:

1. ....
....

2. ....
....

3. ....
....

FEELINGS:

How did you feel today?...

How do you feel now? ....

How do you intend to feel tomorrow? ....

INSPIRATION:

Did you receive inspiration today? ....

Describe what you were inspired to do or say ....
....

FOOD EXPERIMENT:

What single item of food did you experiment with today?............................

Describe how you felt? ....
....

Does your unique body process this food easily? ....

QUOTE OF THE DAY:

" In this reality, nothing is more powerful than thought. The thoughts you think create the life you live. It's as simple as this. It is the fundamental design of the system of physical reality. You are here to practice your powers of creation by choosing thoughts that align with what you want." *Joshua*

Morning Playbook

MEDITATION:

Duration .... Type...

Time of Day .... Satisfaction Level: 1 2 3 4 5 6 7 8 9 10

Notes: ....

....

APPRECIATION:

List 3 things you appreciate about your life:

1. ....

   ....

2. ....

   ....

3. ....

   ....

INTENTIONS:

Set your general intentions for the day:

....

....

....

....

....

....

Evening Playbook

GRATITUDE:

List 3 things you are grateful for (which can include future manifestations):

1. ....

....

2. ....

....

3. ....

....

AFFIRMATIONS:

Write 3 affirmations:

1. ....

....

2. ....

....

3. ....

....

FEELINGS:

How did you feel today? ....

How do you feel now? ....

How do you intend to feel tomorrow? ....

INSPIRATION:

Did you receive inspiration today? ....

Describe what you were inspired to do or say ....

....

FOOD EXPERIMENT:

What single item of food did you experiment with today?................................

Describe how you felt? ....

....

Does your unique body process this food easily? ....

QUOTE OF THE DAY:

66 When you believe that you know how to get from where you are now to the eventual manifestation of your desire, you are attempting to create a reality based on limited information. You think you know how everything should unfold. When things don't turn out as you hoped or expected, you feel negative emotion. You get upset. The reason you are feeling negative emotion is because of fear. When you expect one thing to happen and something else happens instead, you feel fear. You believe that it was wrong to happen this way. However, you really can't imagine how all of this will unfold and so you are simply making it all up." *Joshua*

Morning Playbook

MEDITATION:

Duration .... Type..

Time of Day .... Satisfaction Level: 1 2 3 4 5 6 7 8 9 10

Notes: ....

....

APPRECIATION:

List 3 things you appreciate about your life:

1. ....

....

2. ....

....

3. ....

....

INTENTIONS:

Set your general intentions for the day:

....

....

....

....

....

Evening Playbook

GRATITUDE:

List 3 things you are grateful for (which can include future manifestations):

1. ....
   ....
2. ....
   ....
3. ....
   ....

AFFIRMATIONS:

Write 3 affirmations:

1. ....
   ....
2. ....
   ....
3. ....
   ....

FEELINGS:

How did you feel today? ....

How do you feel now? ....

How do you intend to feel tomorrow? ....

INSPIRATION:

Did you receive inspiration today? ....

Describe what you were inspired to do or say ....
....

FOOD EXPERIMENT:

What single item of food did you experiment with today? ....

Describe how you felt? ....
....

Does your unique body process this food easily? ....

QUOTE OF THE DAY:

" We are here to tell you that your life is like a roller coaster and that is by design. If you knew what was coming, the game would not be any fun. So it's fun not to know what the day will bring. It's fun to explore certain aspects of physical reality. It's fun that things cannot be predicted. When you try to figure out what's going to happen next, well, that's fun too. When you become attached to your predictions, you cause yourself pain when the ride takes an unexpected turn. Release your attachments to your predictions. If things turn out differently than you expected, believe that it's for your highest good." *Joshua*

Morning Playbook

MEDITATION:

Duration ....   Type..

Time of Day ....   Satisfaction Level: 1   2   3   4   5   6   7   8   9   10

Notes: ....

....

APPRECIATION:

List 3 things you appreciate about your life:

1. ....

   ....

2. ....

   ....

3. ....

   ....

INTENTIONS:

Set your general intentions for the day:

....

....

....

....

Evening Playbook

GRATITUDE:

List 3 things you are grateful for (which can include future manifestations):

1. ....
....
2. ....
....
3. ....
....

AFFIRMATIONS:

Write 3 affirmations:

1. ....
....
2. ....
....
3. ....
....

FEELINGS:

How did you feel today? ....

How do you feel now? ....

How do you intend to feel tomorrow? ....

INSPIRATION:

Did you receive inspiration today? ....

Describe what you were inspired to do or say ....

....

FOOD EXPERIMENT:

What single item of food did you experiment with today?.................................

Describe how you felt? ....

....

Does your unique body process this food easily? ....

QUOTE OF THE DAY:

" Did you know that your thoughts control your weight and nothing else? Did you know that you created a perception of who you are and that your thoughts always align with your perception? Did you know you could alter your perception of yourself if you wanted to? It's true. You have created a perception of who you are. Through all your experiences, you've developed a persona. This persona is not real; it's completely imaginary. No one else sees you like you see yourself." *Joshua*

Morning Playbook

MEDITATION:

Duration ....   Type...

Time of Day ....   Satisfaction Level: 1   2   3   4   5   6   7   8   9   10

Notes: ....

....

APPRECIATION:

List 3 things you appreciate about your life:

1. ....

   ....

2. ....

   ....

3. ....

   ....

INTENTIONS:

Set your general intentions for the day:

....

....

....

....

....

....

Evening Playbook

GRATITUDE:

List 3 things you are grateful for (which can include future manifestations):

1. ....
   ....
2. ....
   ....
3. ....
   ....

AFFIRMATIONS:

Write 3 affirmations:

1. ....
   ....
2. ....
   ....
3. ....
   ....

FEELINGS:

How did you feel today?...

How do you feel now?...

How do you intend to feel tomorrow? ....

INSPIRATION:

Did you receive inspiration today? ....

Describe what you were inspired to do or say ....
....

FOOD EXPERIMENT:

What single item of food did you experiment with today?.................................

Describe how you felt? ....
....

Does your unique body process this food easily? ....

QUOTE OF THE DAY:

" Accept your body as it is. Love your body in its present shape. Be comfortable in your body now and then seek to create an improved physical condition. Move toward what you desire and not away from what you dislike. When you understand that your body was created for you alone, you can modify the shape and condition of it through appreciation and acceptance." *Joshua*

Morning Playbook

MEDITATION:

Duration .... Type..

Time of Day .... Satisfaction Level: 1 2 3 4 5 6 7 8 9 10

Notes: ....

....

APPRECIATION:

List 3 things you appreciate about your life:

1. ....

....

2. ....

....

3. ....

....

INTENTIONS:

Set your general intentions for the day:

....

....

....

....

....

....

Evening Playbook

GRATITUDE:

List 3 things you are grateful for (which can include future manifestations):

1. ....

   ....

2. ....

   ....

3. ....

   ....

AFFIRMATIONS:

Write 3 affirmations:

1. ....

   ....

2. ....

   ....

3. ....

   ....

FEELINGS:

How did you feel today? ....

How do you feel now? ....

How do you intend to feel tomorrow? ....

INSPIRATION:

Did you receive inspiration today? ....

Describe what you were inspired to do or say ....

....

FOOD EXPERIMENT:

What single item of food did you experiment with today?...........

Describe how you felt? ....

....

Does your unique body process this food easily? ....

QUOTE OF THE DAY:

" If you can place the focus of your desire on feeling good in your body rather than trying to change how it looks, then you will receive inspiration that will help you create a good-feeling body. When your body feels good, not only will you return to your natural weight and shape, but every cell in your body will be receiving well-being and functioning optimally. You will not only feel good, you will be healthier too. When you feel good and maintain your health, your body will take its natural shape." *Joshua*

Morning Playbook

MEDITATION:

Duration ....   Type...

Time of Day ....   Satisfaction Level: 1   2   3   4   5   6   7   8   9   10

Notes: ....

....

APPRECIATION:

List 3 things you appreciate about your life:

1. ....

   ....

2. ....

   ....

3. ....

   ....

INTENTIONS:

Set your general intentions for the day:

....

....

....

....

....

Evening Playbook

GRATITUDE:

List 3 things you are grateful for (which can include future manifestations):

1. ....
   ....
2. ....
   ....
3. ....
   ....

AFFIRMATIONS:

Write 3 affirmations:

1. ....
   ....
2. ....
   ....
3. ....
   ....

FEELINGS:

How did you feel today? ....

How do you feel now? ....

How do you intend to feel tomorrow? ....

INSPIRATION:

Did you receive inspiration today? ....

Describe what you were inspired to do or say ....
....

FOOD EXPERIMENT:

What single item of food did you experiment with today? ....

Describe how you felt? ....
....

Does your unique body process this food easily? ....

QUOTE OF THE DAY:

❝ If you care about how you feel and your desire is to feel good, you will be guided to foods that match how you want to feel. You will be inspired to choose restaurants and order meals that will make you feel good. You will be interested in new foods. You might read articles, overhear conversations, or receive new thoughts and ideas, all of which will lead you toward your desire. You might receive inspiration to go for a walk after dinner, or to ride a bike, or to take a yoga class, or to play tennis." *Joshua*

Morning Playbook

MEDITATION:

Duration .... Type...

Time of Day .... Satisfaction Level: 1 2 3 4 5 6 7 8 9 10

Notes: ....
....

APPRECIATION:

List 3 things you appreciate about your life:

1. ....
....

2. ....
....

3. ....
....

INTENTIONS:

Set your general intentions for the day:

....
....
....
....
....

Evening Playbook

GRATITUDE:

List 3 things you are grateful for (which can include future manifestations):

1. ....

   ....

2. ....

   ....

3. ....

   ....

AFFIRMATIONS:

Write 3 affirmations:

1. ....

   ....

2. ....

   ....

3. ....

   ....

FEELINGS:

How did you feel today? ....

How do you feel now? ....

How do you intend to feel tomorrow? ....

INSPIRATION:

Did you receive inspiration today? ....

Describe what you were inspired to do or say ....

....

FOOD EXPERIMENT:

What single item of food did you experiment with today?...................................

Describe how you felt? ....

....

Does your unique body process this food easily? ....

QUOTE OF THE DAY:

66 Intention is one of the most powerful tools in the universe. Intention brings your focus onto what is wanted. When you intend for something to happen, the universe understands this within the framework of your vibrational signal. Your focus of attention shines a light on the object of your desire and the universe responds to that. When you intend, you create focus." *Joshua*

Morning Playbook

MEDITATION:

Duration ....   Type...

Time of Day ....   Satisfaction Level: 1   2   3   4   5   6   7   8   9   10

Notes: ....

....

APPRECIATION:

List 3 things you appreciate about your life:

1. ....

....

2. ....

....

3. ....

....

INTENTIONS:

Set your general intentions for the day:

....

....

....

....

....

....

Evening Playbook

GRATITUDE:

List 3 things you are grateful for (which can include future manifestations):

1. ....

   ....

2. ....

   ....

3. ....

   ....

AFFIRMATIONS:

Write 3 affirmations:

1. ....

   ....

2. ....

   ....

3. ....

   ....

FEELINGS:

How did you feel today? ....

How do you feel now? ....

How do you intend to feel tomorrow? ....

INSPIRATION:

Did you receive inspiration today? ....

Describe what you were inspired to do or say ....

....

FOOD EXPERIMENT:

What single item of food did you experiment with today? ....

Describe how you felt? ....

....

Does your unique body process this food easily? ....

QUOTE OF THE DAY:

" Most people believe that in order to feel good, something must happen first. Unfortunately, this simply cannot work in an attractive universe. Unless you feel good first, you cannot receive good-feeling experiences. When you focus on what's wrong in your life and you seek to correct that, ultimately, you will receive more of that." *Joshua*

Morning Playbook

MEDITATION:

Duration .... Type..

Time of Day .... Satisfaction Level: 1   2   3   4   5   6   7   8   9   10

Notes: ....

....

APPRECIATION:

List 3 things you appreciate about your life:

1. ....

....

2. ....

....

3. ....

....

INTENTIONS:

Set your general intentions for the day:

....

....

....

....

....

....

Evening Playbook

GRATITUDE:

List 3 things you are grateful for (which can include future manifestations):

1. ....
....

2. ....
....

3. ....
....

AFFIRMATIONS:

Write 3 affirmations:

1. ....
....

2. ....
....

3. ....
....

FEELINGS:

How did you feel today? ....

How do you feel now? ....

How do you intend to feel tomorrow? ....

INSPIRATION:

Did you receive inspiration today? ....

Describe what you were inspired to do or say ....
....

FOOD EXPERIMENT:

What single item of food did you experiment with today? ....

Describe how you felt? ....
....

Does your unique body process this food easily? ....

QUOTE OF THE DAY:

" Losing weight is like holding up a wall that's about to fall over. You can stand there and prop up the wall for a little while, but eventually you'll become weary and you'll want to do something else. You'll give up and let the wall fall down. You do not have the strength or endurance necessary to keep holding the wall up forever. Sooner or later you'll give up and the wall will come crashing down." *Joshua*

Morning Playbook

MEDITATION:

Duration .... Type...

Time of Day .... Satisfaction Level: 1 2 3 4 5 6 7 8 9 10

Notes: ....

....

APPRECIATION:

List 3 things you appreciate about your life:

1. ....

   ....

2. ....

   ....

3. ....

   ....

INTENTIONS:

Set your general intentions for the day:

....

....

....

....

....

....

Evening Playbook

GRATITUDE:

List 3 things you are grateful for (which can include future manifestations):

1. ....
....
2. ....
....
3. ....
....

AFFIRMATIONS:

Write 3 affirmations:

1. ....
....
2. ....
....
3. ....
....

FEELINGS:

How did you feel today? ....

How do you feel now? ....

How do you intend to feel tomorrow? ....

INSPIRATION:

Did you receive inspiration today? ....

Describe what you were inspired to do or say ....
....

FOOD EXPERIMENT:

What single item of food did you experiment with today? ....

Describe how you felt? ....
....

Does your unique body process this food easily? ....

QUOTE OF THE DAY:

" You are not enjoying the game of losing weight because to you it's a struggle and nothing about it is enjoyable. If it's not enjoyable, don't do it. If you are not inspired to join a gym, don't do it. If you are not inspired to go on some fad diet, don't do it. If you are not inspired to start jogging, don't start. Without the inspiration to do something, the action will not work. There is no gain in pain. Anyone who ever said that got something out of the pain. They enjoyed the pain; you don't have to." *Joshua*

Morning Playbook

MEDITATION:

Duration .... Type...

Time of Day .... Satisfaction Level: 1 2 3 4 5 6 7 8 9 10

Notes: ....

....

APPRECIATION:

List 3 things you appreciate about your life:

1. ....

....

2. ....

....

3. ....

....

INTENTIONS:

Set your general intentions for the day:

....

....

....

....

....

Evening Playbook

GRATITUDE:

List 3 things you are grateful for (which can include future manifestations):

1. ....
....

2. ....
....

3. ....
....

AFFIRMATIONS:

Write 3 affirmations:

1. ....
....

2. ....
....

3. ....
....

FEELINGS:

How did you feel today? ....

How do you feel now? ....

How do you intend to feel tomorrow? ....

INSPIRATION:

Did you receive inspiration today? ....

Describe what you were inspired to do or say ....
....

FOOD EXPERIMENT:

What single item of food did you experiment with today?...............

Describe how you felt? ....
....

Does your unique body process this food easily? ....

QUOTE OF THE DAY:

" Do not take action when you feel bad. Only take action when you feel good. Intend to feel good and you will be inspired to take action that causes you to feel even better." *Joshua*

Morning Playbook

MEDITATION:

Duration .... Type...

Time of Day .... Satisfaction Level: 1 2 3 4 5 6 7 8 9 10

Notes: ....
....
....

APPRECIATION:

List 3 things you appreciate about your life:

1. ....
   ....

2. ....
   ....

3. ....
   ....

INTENTIONS:

Set your general intentions for the day:

....
....
....
....
....
....
....

Evening Playbook

GRATITUDE:

List 3 things you are grateful for (which can include future manifestations):

1. ....

....

2. ....

....

3. ....

....

AFFIRMATIONS:

Write 3 affirmations:

1. ....

....

2. ....

....

3. ....

....

FEELINGS:

How did you feel today? ....

How do you feel now? ....

How do you intend to feel tomorrow? ....

INSPIRATION:

Did you receive inspiration today? ....

Describe what you were inspired to do or say ....

....

FOOD EXPERIMENT:

What single item of food did you experiment with today? ....

Describe how you felt? ....

....

Does your unique body process this food easily? ....

QUOTE OF THE DAY:

❝ Inspiration is exciting, interesting, and makes sense in the moment. If you're feeling good and you receive inspiration to do something, it will seem logical. It will be as if it's something you simply must do. This action will always be for your greatest benefit and highest good. However, if there is fear involved, you might second guess yourself. If you truly feel inspired, you can overcome the fear and take the action anyway. The feeling you receive from taking action in spite of your fear is exhilaration." *Joshua*

Morning Playbook

MEDITATION:

Duration .... Type...

Time of Day .... Satisfaction Level: 1 2 3 4 5 6 7 8 9 10

Notes: ....
....

APPRECIATION:

List 3 things you appreciate about your life:

1. ....
   ....
2. ....
   ....
3. ....
   ....

INTENTIONS:

Set your general intentions for the day:

....
....
....
....
....

Evening Playbook

GRATITUDE:

List 3 things you are grateful for (which can include future manifestations):

1. ....
....

2. ....
....

3. ....
....

AFFIRMATIONS:

Write 3 affirmations:

1. ....
....

2. ....
....

3. ....
....

FEELINGS:

How did you feel today? ....

How do you feel now? ....

How do you intend to feel tomorrow? ....

INSPIRATION:

Did you receive inspiration today? ....

Describe what you were inspired to do or say ....
....

FOOD EXPERIMENT:

What single item of food did you experiment with today? ....

Describe how you felt? ....
....

Does your unique body process this food easily? ....

QUOTE OF THE DAY:

" Everything you want is coming to you. This is the philosophy of a conscious creator. If you want a lean body, then the way to that body is not by doing something drastic like adopting a starvation diet or a painful workout program. The way to receive anything you want, including a lean body, is to allow it to come to you. You can't force it to come. You can't really make it happen. You must allow it to come." *Joshua*

Morning Playbook

MEDITATION:

Duration .... Type...

Time of Day .... Satisfaction Level: 1 2 3 4 5 6 7 8 9 10

Notes: ....

....

APPRECIATION:

List 3 things you appreciate about your life:

1. ....

    ....

2. ....

    ....

3. ....

    ....

INTENTIONS:

Set your general intentions for the day:

....

....

....

....

....

....

Evening Playbook

GRATITUDE:

List 3 things you are grateful for (which can include future manifestations):

1. ....
   ....

2. ....
   ....

3. ....
   ....

AFFIRMATIONS:

Write 3 affirmations:

1. ....
   ....

2. ....
   ....

3. ....
   ....

FEELINGS:

How did you feel today? ....

How do you feel now? ....

How do you intend to feel tomorrow? ....

INSPIRATION:

Did you receive inspiration today? ....

Describe what you were inspired to do or say ....
....

FOOD EXPERIMENT:

What single item of food did you experiment with today? ....

Describe how you felt? ....
....

Does your unique body process this food easily? ....

QUOTE OF THE DAY:

" So many of you want something because you think that having it will solve some other problem. There is only one way to solve any problem. Realize that it's not a problem, it's simply a message. Understand that you can't solve any problems. You can only work on your vibration. When you see something as a problem, you are making it wrong. Since there is no wrong, only points of view, only limited and higher perspectives, only your bias and individual judgment, you cannot remove the thing to solve the problem. All you can do is change. You can change your perspective, your judgment, and your point of view. You change you, not the thing you do not like." —Joshua

Morning Playbook

MEDITATION:

Duration .... Type..

Time of Day .... Satisfaction Level: 1 2 3 4 5 6 7 8 9 10

Notes: ....

....

APPRECIATION:

List 3 things you appreciate about your life:

1. ....

   ....

2. ....

   ....

3. ....

   ....

INTENTIONS:

Set your general intentions for the day:

....

....

....

....

Evening Playbook

GRATITUDE:

List 3 things you are grateful for (which can include future manifestations):

1. ....

....

2. ....

....

3. ....

....

AFFIRMATIONS:

Write 3 affirmations:

1. ....

....

2. ....

....

3. ....

....

FEELINGS:

How did you feel today? ....

How do you feel now? ....

How do you intend to feel tomorrow? ....

INSPIRATION:

Did you receive inspiration today? ....

Describe what you were inspired to do or say ....

....

FOOD EXPERIMENT:

What single item of food did you experiment with today?...................

Describe how you felt? ....

....

Does your unique body process this food easily? ....

QUOTE OF THE DAY:

" When something pops up in your life, it is there for you even when you don't think it is. If it came, it came as a response to your vibration. Everything you want is coming to you. You must be transformed in order for you to see it. Sometimes you hold onto some very limiting beliefs and these thought forms create the illusion that what you want is out of your reach. When you can shift your perception by altering the intensity of these limiting beliefs, suddenly the illusion is removed." *Joshua*

Morning Playbook

MEDITATION:

Duration ....   Type..

Time of Day ....   Satisfaction Level: 1 2 3 4 5 6 7 8 9 10

Notes: ....

....

APPRECIATION:

List 3 things you appreciate about your life:

1. ....

....

2. ....

....

3. ....

....

INTENTIONS:

Set your general intentions for the day:

....

....

....

....

....

Evening Playbook

GRATITUDE:

List 3 things you are grateful for (which can include future manifestations):

1. ....
....

2. ....
....

3. ....
....

AFFIRMATIONS:

Write 3 affirmations:

1. ....
....

2. ....
....

3. ....
....

FEELINGS:

How did you feel today? ....

How do you feel now? ....

How do you intend to feel tomorrow? ....

INSPIRATION:

Did you receive inspiration today? ....

Describe what you were inspired to do or say ....
....

FOOD EXPERIMENT:

What single item of food did you experiment with today? ....

Describe how you felt? ....
....

Does your unique body process this food easily? ....

QUOTE OF THE DAY:

❝ When you accept the conditions as they are, you are agreeing with the design of the universe. You understand that the conditions have been created to support whatever it is you came here to explore. You know that your body is part of that exploration and that it is perfect as it is because it is allowing you to explore reality in the way you intended. If you look at any aspect of it and think it's inadequate, then you cannot trust that this is all for you. You are either a conscious creator and believe that this is all part of the process of expansion and growth and you take responsibility for your creation, or you must perceive yourself as a victim without any responsibility." *Joshua*

Morning Playbook

MEDITATION:

Duration ....   Type...

Time of Day ....   Satisfaction Level: 1   2   3   4   5   6   7   8   9   10

Notes: ....

....

APPRECIATION:

List 3 things you appreciate about your life:

1. ....

   ....

2. ....

   ....

3. ....

   ....

INTENTIONS:

Set your general intentions for the day:

....

....

....

....

Evening Playbook

GRATITUDE:

List 3 things you are grateful for (which can include future manifestations):

1. ....
....

2. ....
....

3. ....
....

AFFIRMATIONS:

Write 3 affirmations:

1. ....
....

2. ....
....

3. ....
....

FEELINGS:

How did you feel today? ....

How do you feel now? ....

How do you intend to feel tomorrow? ....

INSPIRATION:

Did you receive inspiration today? ....

Describe what you were inspired to do or say ....
....

FOOD EXPERIMENT:

What single item of food did you experiment with today?................................

Describe how you felt? ....
....

Does your unique body process this food easily? ....

QUOTE OF THE DAY:

" If you have a health problem, a financial issue, an addiction, or any other unwanted condition, it all stems from resistance to some aspect of your life that you willingly and intentionally came here to explore. By attempting to remove the inner feeling with an outer action, you create dissonance. You are simply attempting to avoid the thing by calling it wrong." *Joshua*

Morning Playbook

MEDITATION:

Duration .... Type...

Time of Day .... Satisfaction Level: 1 2 3 4 5 6 7 8 9 10

Notes: ....
....
....

APPRECIATION:

List 3 things you appreciate about your life:

1. ....
....

2. ....
....

3. ....
....

INTENTIONS:

Set your general intentions for the day:

....
....
....
....
....
....

Evening Playbook

List 3 things you are grateful for (which can include future manifestations):

1. ....

....

2. ....

....

3. ....

....

AFFIRMATIONS:

Write 3 affirmations:

1. ....

....

2. ....

....

3. ....

....

FEELINGS:

How did you feel today? ....

How do you feel now? ....

How do you intend to feel tomorrow? ....

INSPIRATION:

Did you receive inspiration today? ....

Describe what you were inspired to do or say ....

....

FOOD EXPERIMENT:

What single item of food did you experiment with today?..................................

Describe how you felt? ....

....

Does your unique body process this food easily? ....

QUOTE OF THE DAY:

❝ Pain is self-inflicted. You shy away from situations that might give rise to negative emotion because you fear the pain associated with these emotions. In doing so, you are not confronting the issue at hand. In order to get what you truly want, in order to live life on your terms, you must move through the issue that presents itself." *Joshua*

Morning Playbook

MEDITATION:

Duration ....   Type...

Time of Day ....   Satisfaction Level: 1 2 3 4 5 6 7 8 9 10

Notes: ....

....

APPRECIATION:

List 3 things you appreciate about your life:

1. ....

   ....

2. ....

   ....

3. ....

   ....

INTENTIONS:

Set your general intentions for the day:

....

....

....

....

....

....

Evening Playbook

GRATITUDE:

List 3 things you are grateful for (which can include future manifestations):

1. ....
....
2. ....
....
3. ....
....

AFFIRMATIONS:

Write 3 affirmations:

1. ....
....
2. ....
....
3. ....
....

FEELINGS:

How did you feel today? ....

How do you feel now? ....

How do you intend to feel tomorrow? ....

INSPIRATION:

Did you receive inspiration today? ....

Describe what you were inspired to do or say ....
....

FOOD EXPERIMENT:

What single item of food did you experiment with today? ....

Describe how you felt? ....
....

Does your unique body process this food easily? ....

QUOTE OF THE DAY:

" The concept that there is no wrong anywhere in the universe is what allowing is all about. If there is no wrong, there is no resistance. If you perceive everything as right, you are an allower. Without resistance, you can move easily from the vibration you are emitting right now, which is creating the life you are currently living, to a new and higher vibration that will create the life you prefer." *Joshua*

Morning Playbook

MEDITATION:

Duration ....   Type...

Time of Day ....   Satisfaction Level: 1   2   3   4   5   6   7   8   9   10

Notes: ....

....

APPRECIATION:

List 3 things you appreciate about your life:

1. ....

   ....

2. ....

   ....

3. ....

   ....

INTENTIONS:

Set your general intentions for the day:

....

....

....

....

....

....

Evening Playbook

GRATITUDE:

List 3 things you are grateful for (which can include future manifestations):

1. ....
....

2. ....
....

3. ....
....

AFFIRMATIONS:

Write 3 affirmations:

1. ....
....

2. ....
....

3. ....
....

FEELINGS:

How did you feel today? ....

How do you feel now? ....

How do you intend to feel tomorrow? ....

INSPIRATION:

Did you receive inspiration today? ....

Describe what you were inspired to do or say ....
....

FOOD EXPERIMENT:

What single item of food did you experiment with today?........................

Describe how you felt? ....
....

Does your unique body process this food easily? ....

QUOTE OF THE DAY:

" Your desire creates the need to alter your vibration. If you had no desires, if you were perfectly content, you would feel no resistance. You would experience no negative emotion. However, since you have birthed a desire, the universe is answering your request. You do not match whatever it is you want and therefore you must be changed. If your desire is to come to you, you must become a match to it. It's as simple as that." *Joshua*

Morning Playbook

MEDITATION:

Duration ....   Type...

Time of Day ....   Satisfaction Level: 1   2   3   4   5   6   7   8   9   10

Notes: ....

....

APPRECIATION:

List 3 things you appreciate about your life:

1. ....

....

2. ....

....

3. ....

....

INTENTIONS:

Set your general intentions for the day:

....

....

....

....

....

....

Evening Playbook

GRATITUDE:

List 3 things you are grateful for (which can include future manifestations):

1. ....
....
2. ....
....
3. ....
....

AFFIRMATIONS:

Write 3 affirmations:

1. ....
....
2. ....
....
3. ....
....

FEELINGS:

How did you feel today? ....

How do you feel now? ....

How do you intend to feel tomorrow? ....

INSPIRATION:

Did you receive inspiration today? ....

Describe what you were inspired to do or say ....
....

FOOD EXPERIMENT:

What single item of food did you experiment with today? ....

Describe how you felt? ....
....

Does your unique body process this food easily? ....

QUOTE OF THE DAY:

" If you allow the changes to your beliefs to be made, you will easily become a match to that which you want. If you resist any change to your belief system, you will feel negative emotion. The negative emotion need not be painful; it's simply a message letting you know that you are resisting the change you want. If you can release your limiting beliefs, you will remove the barrier that separates you from your desire. That is all that is going on here." *Joshua*

Morning Playbook

MEDITATION:

Duration ....   Type...

Time of Day ....   Satisfaction Level: 1 2 3 4 5 6 7 8 9 10

Notes: ....
....

APPRECIATION:

List 3 things you appreciate about your life:

1. ....
   ....

2. ....
   ....

3. ....
   ....

INTENTIONS:

Set your general intentions for the day:

....
....
....
....
....
....

Evening Playbook

GRATITUDE:

List 3 things you are grateful for (which can include future manifestations):

1. ....
   ....

2. ....
   ....

3. ....
   ....

AFFIRMATIONS:

Write 3 affirmations:

1. ....
   ....

2. ....
   ....

3. ....
   ....

FEELINGS:

How did you feel today? ....

How do you feel now? ....

How do you intend to feel tomorrow? ....

INSPIRATION:

Did you receive inspiration today? ....

Describe what you were inspired to do or say ....
....

FOOD EXPERIMENT:

What single item of food did you experiment with today?..........

Describe how you felt? ....
....

Does your unique body process this food easily? ....

QUOTE OF THE DAY:

66 Allowing is the acknowledgment that everything that shows up in your life is for your benefit, whether it seems like it or not. You might judge it as bad, but that is just resistance. It is good. If you can see it as progress toward that which you want, then you are an allower. If you choose to hang on to your limiting beliefs and suffer through the negative emotion that comes with resistance, then that too is your choice. Chose to allow limiting beliefs to fade and you will receive all that you want. Resist any challenge to your limiting beliefs and not only will you prevent your desire from being manifested in your reality, but you'll also experience continued negative emotion." *Joshua*

Morning Playbook

MEDITATION:

Duration .... Type..

Time of Day .... Satisfaction Level: 1   2   3   4   5   6   7   8   9   10

Notes: ....

....

APPRECIATION:

List 3 things you appreciate about your life:

1. ....

   ....

2. ....

   ....

3. ....

   ....

INTENTIONS:

Set your general intentions for the day:

....

....

....

....

Evening Playbook

GRATITUDE:

List 3 things you are grateful for (which can include future manifestations):

1. ....
   ....
2. ....
   ....
3. ....
   ....

AFFIRMATIONS:

Write 3 affirmations:

1. ....
   ....
2. ....
   ....
3. ....
   ....

FEELINGS:

How did you feel today? ....

How do you feel now? ....

How do you intend to feel tomorrow? ....

INSPIRATION:

Did you receive inspiration today? ....

Describe what you were inspired to do or say ....

....

FOOD EXPERIMENT:

What single item of food did you experiment with today? ....

Describe how you felt? ....

....

Does your unique body process this food easily? ....

QUOTE OF THE DAY:

" When you are focused on feeling good, inspiration is always striking. You receive thoughts and when you follow them, they will lead to people, places, and events that will move you toward that which you desire. These thoughts may lead you right into a manifestation event that will challenge your beliefs. This could be painful if you resist it, but when you understand what's going on, there's no need for emotional pain or resistance. This is a chance to alter some of your limiting beliefs. Once you've done that, you are another step closer to realizing a dream." *Joshua*

Morning Playbook

MEDITATION:

Duration .... Type...

Time of Day .... Satisfaction Level: 1 2 3 4 5 6 7 8 9 10

Notes: ....

....

APPRECIATION:

List 3 things you appreciate about your life:

1. ....

....

2. ....

....

3. ....

....

INTENTIONS:

Set your general intentions for the day:

....

....

....

....

....

Evening Playbook

GRATITUDE:

List 3 things you are grateful for (which can include future manifestations):

1. ....
....

2. ....
....

3. ....
....

AFFIRMATIONS:

Write 3 affirmations:

1. ....
....

2. ....
....

3. ....
....

FEELINGS:

How did you feel today? ....

How do you feel now? ....

How do you intend to feel tomorrow? ....

INSPIRATION:

Did you receive inspiration today? ....

Describe what you were inspired to do or say ....
....

FOOD EXPERIMENT:

What single item of food did you experiment with today?...

Describe how you felt? ....
....

Does your unique body process this food easily? ....

QUOTE OF THE DAY:

" When you hear about a new diet and how it's worked for many people, what is happening is a mass shift of beliefs. People who believe that something is working temporarily enter the state of allowing and come into vibration range of the thing they want. They use their belief in this new diet to cause themselves to suspend their limiting beliefs, if only for a little while. And it works as long as their limiting beliefs remain low in intensity. However, as soon as their limiting beliefs come back, their weight returns." *Joshua*

Morning Playbook

MEDITATION:

Duration ....   Type...

Time of Day ....   Satisfaction Level: 1 2 3 4 5 6 7 8 9 10

Notes: ....

....

APPRECIATION:

List 3 things you appreciate about your life:

1. ....

....

2. ....

....

3. ....

....

INTENTIONS:

Set your general intentions for the day:

....

....

....

....

....

Evening Playbook

GRATITUDE:

List 3 things you are grateful for (which can include future manifestations):

1. ....

....

2. ....

....

3. ....

....

AFFIRMATIONS:

Write 3 affirmations:

1. ....

....

2. ....

....

3. ....

....

FEELINGS:

How did you feel today? ....

How do you feel now? ....

How do you intend to feel tomorrow? ....

INSPIRATION:

Did you receive inspiration today? ....

Describe what you were inspired to do or say ....

....

FOOD EXPERIMENT:

What single item of food did you experiment with today? ....

Describe how you felt? ....

....

Does your unique body process this food easily? ....

QUOTE OF THE DAY:

" The more you are open to the idea of experimentation, the more you will find it easier to dismiss your fears. Fear arises at the moment of inspiration because you start to think of all the things that could go wrong. You believe in the possibility of failure. There is no failure, there is only experience and all experience is valid and valuable. If you think to yourself, "This is just an experiment and I'm here on a mission of discovery," then you cannot fail. Experimentation removes the possibility of failure." *Joshua*

Morning Playbook

MEDITATION:

Duration .... Type..

Time of Day .... Satisfaction Level: 1 2 3 4 5 6 7 8 9 10

Notes: ....

....

APPRECIATION:

List 3 things you appreciate about your life:

1. ....

....

2. ....

....

3. ....

....

INTENTIONS:

Set your general intentions for the day:

....

....

....

....

....

Evening Playbook

GRATITUDE:

List 3 things you are grateful for (which can include future manifestations):

1. ....

....

2. ....

....

3. ....

....

AFFIRMATIONS:

Write 3 affirmations:

1. ....

....

2. ....

....

3. ....

....

FEELINGS:

How did you feel today? ....

How do you feel now? ....

How do you intend to feel tomorrow? ....

INSPIRATION:

Did you receive inspiration today? ....

Describe what you were inspired to do or say ....

....

FOOD EXPERIMENT:

What single item of food did you experiment with today? ....

Describe how you felt? ....

....

Does your unique body process this food easily? ....

QUOTE OF THE DAY:

❝ There is no such thing as failure. To redefine the word failure, you might call it an ""unexpected outcome for which I am using a limited perspective to judge the results."" From the higher perspective, you cannot fail, because all experience further defines your desires and thus clarifies and focuses your attention to what is wanted." *Joshua*

Morning Playbook

MEDITATION:

Duration ....   Type...

Time of Day ....   Satisfaction Level: 1   2   3   4   5   6   7   8   9   10

Notes: ....

....

APPRECIATION:

List 3 things you appreciate about your life:

1. ....

   ....

2. ....

   ....

3. ....

   ....

INTENTIONS:

Set your general intentions for the day:

....

....

....

....

....

Evening Playbook

GRATITUDE:

List 3 things you are grateful for (which can include future manifestations):

1. ....
....

2. ....
....

3. ....
....

AFFIRMATIONS:

Write 3 affirmations:

1. ....
....

2. ....
....

3. ....
....

FEELINGS:

How did you feel today? ....

How do you feel now? ....

How do you intend to feel tomorrow? ....

INSPIRATION:

Did you receive inspiration today? ....

Describe what you were inspired to do or say ....
....

FOOD EXPERIMENT:

What single item of food did you experiment with today?...............................

Describe how you felt? ....
....

Does your unique body process this food easily? ....

QUOTE OF THE DAY:

" Bring yourself out of your comfort prison and try new things. Do not fear failure. Do not fear the alteration of your persona. Do not fear change. You must change your approach to life, your perception of reality, and who you are being in order to receive anything you desire. If you want something and it does not exist in your life now, you will literally have to change in order for it to enter your reality. You change to match the thing you want and the thing you want will come to you. This is the Law of Attraction." *Joshua*

Morning Playbook

MEDITATION:

Duration .... Type...

Time of Day .... Satisfaction Level: 1 2 3 4 5 6 7 8 9 10

Notes: ....

....

APPRECIATION:

List 3 things you appreciate about your life:

1. ....

....

2. ....

....

3. ....

....

INTENTIONS:

Set your general intentions for the day:

....

....

....

....

....

Evening Playbook

GRATITUDE:

List 3 things you are grateful for (which can include future manifestations):

1. ....
   ....
2. ....
   ....
3. ....
   ....

AFFIRMATIONS:

Write 3 affirmations:

1. ....
   ....
2. ....
   ....
3. ....
   ....

FEELINGS:

How did you feel today? ....

How do you feel now? ....

How do you intend to feel tomorrow? ....

INSPIRATION:

Did you receive inspiration today? ....

Describe what you were inspired to do or say ....
....

FOOD EXPERIMENT:

What single item of food did you experiment with today? ....

Describe how you felt? ....
....

Does your unique body process this food easily? ....

QUOTE OF THE DAY:

" The old approach to life is the one you were taught at a very early age. It is the one where you must change anything you think is bad or wrong. It's the approach where you fight against the conditions you don't like. Where you eradicate anything that seems unpleasant. Where you avoid any condition or situation where there might be a possibility of experiencing negative emotion. Where you hide your feelings and soothe yourself by reacting to the outside conditions. Where you believe that you are a victim of fate and that you really have no control over your life. Where you take no responsibility for the things that appear in your reality." *Joshua*

Morning Playbook

MEDITATION:

Duration .... Type...

Time of Day .... Satisfaction Level: 1 2 3 4 5 6 7 8 9 10

Notes: ....

....

APPRECIATION:

List 3 things you appreciate about your life:

1. ....

....

2. ....

....

3. ....

....

INTENTIONS:

Set your general intentions for the day:

....

....

....

....

Evening Playbook

GRATITUDE:

List 3 things you are grateful for (which can include future manifestations):

1. ....
....

2. ....
....

3. ....
....

AFFIRMATIONS:

Write 3 affirmations:

1. ....
....

2. ....
....

3. ....
....

FEELINGS:

How did you feel today? ....

How do you feel now? ....

How do you intend to feel tomorrow? ....

INSPIRATION:

Did you receive inspiration today? ....

Describe what you were inspired to do or say ....
....

FOOD EXPERIMENT:

What single item of food did you experiment with today? ....

Describe how you felt? ....
....

Does your unique body process this food easily? ....

QUOTE OF THE DAY:

" The radically new approach to life is one of allowing. You understand that you create your own reality and you take responsibility for and pride in your own creation. You understand that you are worthy and unique. You realize that there are no accidents, fate, or coincidences. You understand that everything is right and anything judged as wrong is done so only from a limited perspective. You know that from the higher perspective, everything is right the way it is. You understand that everything is always working out for you. This isn't just a comforting phrase; it is the design of physical reality and can be no other way." *Joshua*

Morning Playbook

MEDITATION:

Duration .... Type..

Time of Day .... Satisfaction Level: 1 2 3 4 5 6 7 8 9 10

Notes: ....

....

APPRECIATION:

List 3 things you appreciate about your life:

1. ....

   ....

2. ....

   ....

3. ....

   ....

INTENTIONS:

Set your general intentions for the day:

....

....

....

....

Evening Playbook

GRATITUDE:

List 3 things you are grateful for (which can include future manifestations):

1. ....
....

2. ....
....

3. ....
....

AFFIRMATIONS:

Write 3 affirmations:

1. ....
....

2. ....
....

3. ....
....

FEELINGS:

How did you feel today? ....

How do you feel now? ....

How do you intend to feel tomorrow? ....

INSPIRATION:

Did you receive inspiration today? ....

Describe what you were inspired to do or say ....
....

FOOD EXPERIMENT:

What single item of food did you experiment with today?...........................

Describe how you felt? ....
....

Does your unique body process this food easily? ....

QUOTE OF THE DAY:

66 Along the way your resistant thoughts influenced your body away from its natural state of health, well-being, and vitality. If you feel a lack of energy, it's due to your resistant thoughts and limiting beliefs. If you have gained weight, it's due to the thoughts you consistently think. If you have a chronic physical ailment, it's because you have a chronic pattern of resistant thought. If your body is addicted to something, it has only to do with your addictive habit of thought. Your body (and your reality) match how and what you are thinking. Change your body by changing the way you think." *Joshua*

Morning Playbook

MEDITATION:

Duration .... Type...

Time of Day .... Satisfaction Level: 1 2 3 4 5 6 7 8 9 10

Notes: ....

....

APPRECIATION:

List 3 things you appreciate about your life:

1. ....

....

2. ....

....

3. ....

....

INTENTIONS:

Set your general intentions for the day:

....

....

....

....

Evening Playbook

GRATITUDE:

List 3 things you are grateful for (which can include future manifestations):

1. ....
....

2. ....
....

3. ....
....

AFFIRMATIONS:

Write 3 affirmations:

1. ....
....

2. ....
....

3. ....
....

FEELINGS:

How did you feel today? ....

How do you feel now? ....

How do you intend to feel tomorrow? ....

INSPIRATION:

Did you receive inspiration today? ....

Describe what you were inspired to do or say ....
....

FOOD EXPERIMENT:

What single item of food did you experiment with today?...................................

Describe how you felt? ....
....

Does your unique body process this food easily? ....

QUOTE OF THE DAY:

“ You have a certain belief about food that is based mostly on bad advice. You have been told that every body is similar and that what is good for one is good (or bad) for all. This is not true. The fundamental truth is that you are unique and so is everyone else. This is quite obvious. So then, if you are unique, wouldn't it make sense that what's good for you may not be good for others and vice versa? What works for you is for you and what works for others is for them." *Joshua*

Morning Playbook

MEDITATION:

Duration ....   Type..

Time of Day ....   Satisfaction Level: 1 2 3 4 5 6 7 8 9 10

Notes: ....

....

APPRECIATION:

List 3 things you appreciate about your life:

1. ....

....

2. ....

....

3. ....

....

INTENTIONS:

Set your general intentions for the day:

....

....

....

....

....

....

Evening Playbook

GRATITUDE:

List 3 things you are grateful for (which can include future manifestations):

1. ....

....

2. ....

....

3. ....

....

AFFIRMATIONS:

Write 3 affirmations:

1. ....

....

2. ....

....

3. ....

....

FEELINGS:

How did you feel today? ....

How do you feel now? ....

How do you intend to feel tomorrow? ....

INSPIRATION:

Did you receive inspiration today? ....

Describe what you were inspired to do or say ....

....

FOOD EXPERIMENT:

What single item of food did you experiment with today?................................

Describe how you felt? ....

....

Does your unique body process this food easily? ....

QUOTE OF THE DAY:

" You do not eat the same food as your dog or cat. You can easily see that they are very different than you. However, just as your dog is different, so is your neighbor, your friend, and your parent. What works for them has nothing to do with what works for you. You are unique. Treat everything you eat as a unique combination of your vibration and its vibration. Determine for yourself what works and what doesn't. Do not blindly accept that some foods are good and others are bad. If your body is not currently at its natural shape, it's because your belief about the foods you are eating must be challenged." *Joshua*

Morning Playbook

MEDITATION:

Duration .... Type...

Time of Day .... Satisfaction Level: 1 2 3 4 5 6 7 8 9 10

Notes: ....
....

APPRECIATION:

List 3 things you appreciate about your life:

1. ....
....

2. ....
....

3. ....
....

INTENTIONS:

Set your general intentions for the day:

....
....
....
....
....

Evening Playbook

GRATITUDE:

List 3 things you are grateful for (which can include future manifestations):

1. ....
....

2. ....
....

3. ....
....

AFFIRMATIONS:

Write 3 affirmations:

1. ....
....

2. ....
....

3. ....
....

FEELINGS:

How did you feel today? ....

How do you feel now? ....

How do you intend to feel tomorrow? ....

INSPIRATION:

Did you receive inspiration today? ....

Describe what you were inspired to do or say ....
....

FOOD EXPERIMENT:

What single item of food did you experiment with today?...........................

Describe how you felt? ....
....

Does your unique body process this food easily? ....

QUOTE OF THE DAY:

" Your vibration is unique, so it does not matter what others think or believe. What is good for you is due to a unique combination of your vibration and the vibration of whatever food you eat. You are unique and so that interaction is always unique. If you feel good after eating or drinking something, if you have energy and vitality, then you can know that the food works with your body in a way that is beneficial. If you feel bad, sluggish, constipated, bloated, gassy, etc., then you know that the food is not being easily absorbed into your body." *Joshua*

Morning Playbook

MEDITATION:

Duration ....   Type...

Time of Day ....   Satisfaction Level: 1 2 3 4 5 6 7 8 9 10

Notes: ....

....

APPRECIATION:

List 3 things you appreciate about your life:

1. ....

   ....

2. ....

   ....

3. ....

   ....

INTENTIONS:

Set your general intentions for the day:

....

....

....

....

....

Evening Playbook

GRATITUDE:

List 3 things you are grateful for (which can include future manifestations):

1. ....
....
2. ....
....
3. ....
....

AFFIRMATIONS:

Write 3 affirmations:

1. ....
....
2. ....
....
3. ....
....

FEELINGS:

How did you feel today? ....

How do you feel now? ....

How do you intend to feel tomorrow? ....

INSPIRATION:

Did you receive inspiration today? ....

Describe what you were inspired to do or say ....
....

FOOD EXPERIMENT:

What single item of food did you experiment with today?..............

Describe how you felt? ....
....

Does your unique body process this food easily? ....

QUOTE OF THE DAY:

❝ Experimentation is a device you can use to test the strength of your beliefs. Right now you have a set of beliefs about food that plays a critical role in which foods you will and will not eat. Your body is a representation of your beliefs about the foods you eat. You may be eating or avoiding foods based on your beliefs. Your body's current state is a result of your current set of beliefs. Alter those beliefs and the shape and condition of your body will change." *Joshua*

Morning Playbook

MEDITATION:

Duration .... Type...

Time of Day .... Satisfaction Level: 1 2 3 4 5 6 7 8 9 10

Notes: ....

....

APPRECIATION:

List 3 things you appreciate about your life:

1. ....

   ....

2. ....

   ....

3. ....

   ....

INTENTIONS:

Set your general intentions for the day:

....

....

....

....

....

....

Evening Playbook

GRATITUDE:

List 3 things you are grateful for (which can include future manifestations):

1. ....
....

2. ....
....

3. ....
....

AFFIRMATIONS:

Write 3 affirmations:

1. ....
....

2. ....
....

3. ....
....

FEELINGS:

How did you feel today? ....

How do you feel now? ....

How do you intend to feel tomorrow? ....

INSPIRATION:

Did you receive inspiration today? ....

Describe what you were inspired to do or say ....
....

FOOD EXPERIMENT:

What single item of food did you experiment with today?...................

Describe how you felt? ....
....

Does your unique body process this food easily? ....

QUOTE OF THE DAY:

" If you believe that a certain food is good, it is good for you. If you believe it is bad, then it is bad for you. However, you have never really experimented with most of the foods you eat on a regular basis. You simply assume that some things are good and others are bad. Until you experiment with your own body, we will submit to you that your limiting beliefs about those foods are false. Experiment to find out the truth about food for yourself and as a result, the beliefs that were created through experimentation will be highly beneficial." *Joshua*

Morning Playbook

MEDITATION:

Duration .... Type...

Time of Day .... Satisfaction Level: 1 2 3 4 5 6 7 8 9 10

Notes: ....

....

APPRECIATION:

List 3 things you appreciate about your life:

1. ....

....

2. ....

....

3. ....

....

INTENTIONS:

Set your general intentions for the day:

....

....

....

....

....

Evening Playbook

GRATITUDE:
List 3 things you are grateful for (which can include future manifestations):

1. ....
....

2. ....
....

3. ....
....

AFFIRMATIONS:
Write 3 affirmations:

1. ....
....

2. ....
....

3. ....
....

FEELINGS:
How did you feel today? ....

How do you feel now? ....

How do you intend to feel tomorrow? ....

INSPIRATION:
Did you receive inspiration today? ....

Describe what you were inspired to do or say ....
....

FOOD EXPERIMENT:
What single item of food did you experiment with today?.................

Describe how you felt? ....
....

Does your unique body process this food easily? ....

QUOTE OF THE DAY:

" If you can understand that it is your perception of reality that affects your health, your weight, your relationships, your wealth, and everything else, you can form a more empowering perception by looking at life in a new way. When you understand that everything happens for your benefit, you can allow the lingering effects of negative emotion to fade away. As soon as you can get our premise that nothing you want is achieved but that everything you want is received, you can switch your approach to life from one of trying and efforting, to one of feeling and allowing." *Joshua*

Morning Playbook

MEDITATION:

Duration .... Type..

Time of Day .... Satisfaction Level: 1 2 3 4 5 6 7 8 9 10

Notes: ....

....

APPRECIATION:

List 3 things you appreciate about your life:

1. ....

   ....

2. ....

   ....

3. ....

   ....

INTENTIONS:

Set your general intentions for the day:

....

....

....

....

Evening Playbook

GRATITUDE:

List 3 things you are grateful for (which can include future manifestations):

1. ....
....

2. ....
....

3. ....
....

AFFIRMATIONS:

Write 3 affirmations:

1. ....
....

2. ....
....

3. ....
....

FEELINGS:

How did you feel today? ....

How do you feel now? ....

How do you intend to feel tomorrow? ....

INSPIRATION:

Did you receive inspiration today? ....

Describe what you were inspired to do or say ....
....

FOOD EXPERIMENT:

What single item of food did you experiment with today?.....................

Describe how you felt? ....
....

Does your unique body process this food easily? ....

QUOTE OF THE DAY:

" You are perfect as you are. You chose to explore life in the way you are exploring it. Everything is right. Everything has turned out perfectly. You are perfect as you are. We know this to be true. Any fault you see in yourself is not a fault at all. There is nothing wrong with you because there is no wrong anywhere in the universe. You are perfectly right in every single way. You are good." *Joshua*

Morning Playbook

MEDITATION:

Duration ....   Type..

Time of Day ....   Satisfaction Level: 1 2 3 4 5 6 7 8 9 10

Notes: ....

....

APPRECIATION:

List 3 things you appreciate about your life:

1. ....

....

2. ....

....

3. ....

....

INTENTIONS:

Set your general intentions for the day:

....

....

....

....

....

....

Evening Playbook

GRATITUDE:

List 3 things you are grateful for (which can include future manifestations):

1. ....
....

2. ....
....

3. ....
....

AFFIRMATIONS:

Write 3 affirmations:

1. ....
....

2. ....
....

3. ....
....

FEELINGS:

How did you feel today? ....

How do you feel now? ....

How do you intend to feel tomorrow? ....

INSPIRATION:

Did you receive inspiration today? ....

Describe what you were inspired to do or say ....
....

FOOD EXPERIMENT:

What single item of food did you experiment with today? ....

Describe how you felt? ....
....

Does your unique body process this food easily? ....

QUOTE OF THE DAY:

" The lean body you desire, the abundance you desire, and the relationships you desire all start with love of self. It is good and right to love yourself. You are meant to love yourself above all others. To love yourself is to love others. The two ideas are unified. They are inseparable. You cannot truly love another more than your capacity to love yourself. If you love another truly, then you love yourself truly as well." *Joshua*

Morning Playbook

MEDITATION:

Duration ....   Type..

Time of Day ....   Satisfaction Level: 1   2   3   4   5   6   7   8   9   10

Notes: ....

....

APPRECIATION:

List 3 things you appreciate about your life:

1. ....

   ....

2. ....

   ....

3. ....

   ....

INTENTIONS:

Set your general intentions for the day:

....

....

....

....

....

....

Evening Playbook

GRATITUDE:

List 3 things you are grateful for (which can include future manifestations):

1. ....
....

2. ....
....

3. ....
....

AFFIRMATIONS:

Write 3 affirmations:

1. ....
....

2. ....
....

3. ....
....

FEELINGS:

How did you feel today? ....

How do you feel now? ....

How do you intend to feel tomorrow? ....

INSPIRATION:

Did you receive inspiration today? ....

Describe what you were inspired to do or say ....
....

FOOD EXPERIMENT:

What single item of food did you experiment with today? ....

Describe how you felt? ....
....

Does your unique body process this food easily? ....

QUOTE OF THE DAY:

" When you feel stress, you look for something to improve how you are feeling. You think this is an effective remedy from what you have learned about dealing with stress. The stress is mild and the cure seems easy enough. Just find something, anything, to distract you from how you are feeling. But whenever you look outside yourself to fill that feeling of dread, you are simply affixing a temporary patch. As soon as your mind returns from the distraction, you start to fret and worry all over again. The stress always returns." *Joshua*

Morning Playbook

MEDITATION:

Duration ....   Type...

Time of Day ....   Satisfaction Level: 1   2   3   4   5   6   7   8   9   10

Notes: ....

....

APPRECIATION:

List 3 things you appreciate about your life:

1. ....

   ....

2. ....

   ....

3. ....

   ....

INTENTIONS:

Set your general intentions for the day:

....

....

....

....

....

Evening Playbook

GRATITUDE:

List 3 things you are grateful for (which can include future manifestations):

1. ....
....

2. ....
....

3. ....
....

AFFIRMATIONS:

Write 3 affirmations:

1. ....
....

2. ....
....

3. ....
....

FEELINGS:

How did you feel today? ....

How do you feel now? ....

How do you intend to feel tomorrow? ....

INSPIRATION:

Did you receive inspiration today? ....

Describe what you were inspired to do or say ....
....

FOOD EXPERIMENT:

What single item of food did you experiment with today? ....

Describe how you felt? ....
....

Does your unique body process this food easily? ....

QUOTE OF THE DAY:

" If you were a vibrational match to weighing four hundred pounds, you would have a very specific set of beliefs and feelings about yourself and the world around you. You would look at yourself differently in all areas of your life. You would have a certain specific set of very intense feelings about yourself. You could not weigh four hundred pounds unless you were a vibrational, emotional, and mental match to it." *Joshua*

Morning Playbook

MEDITATION:

Duration .... Type...

Time of Day .... Satisfaction Level: 1 2 3 4 5 6 7 8 9 10

Notes: ....
....

APPRECIATION:

List 3 things you appreciate about your life:

1. ....
   ....
2. ....
   ....
3. ....
   ....

INTENTIONS:

Set your general intentions for the day:

....
....
....
....
....
....

Evening Playbook

GRATITUDE:

List 3 things you are grateful for (which can include future manifestations):

1. ....

....

2. ....

....

3. ....

....

AFFIRMATIONS:

Write 3 affirmations:

1. ....

....

2. ....

....

3. ....

....

FEELINGS:

How did you feel today? ....

How do you feel now? ....

How do you intend to feel tomorrow? ....

INSPIRATION:

Did you receive inspiration today? ....

Describe what you were inspired to do or say ....

....

FOOD EXPERIMENT:

What single item of food did you experiment with today? ....

Describe how you felt? ....

....

Does your unique body process this food easily? ....

QUOTE OF THE DAY:

" Imagine that you knew you were taken care of and that everything would always work out for you. Imagine that you could do no wrong. Imagine that it was not possible for anything to go wrong. Imagine that if something seemed to go wrong that it wasn't wrong at all, but actually it was very good indeed. It's just that from your perspective, you were unable to really see the good that would come of it. Imagine you were safe and always loved. Imagine that you could not fail. If this was the case, then you could not feel fear. If this was true, then you could not worry and without worry or negative emotion, you would not be stressed." *Joshua*

Morning Playbook

MEDITATION:

Duration .... Type...

Time of Day .... Satisfaction Level: 1 2 3 4 5 6 7 8 9 10

Notes: ....

....

APPRECIATION:

List 3 things you appreciate about your life:

1. ....

   ....

2. ....

   ....

3. ....

   ....

INTENTIONS:

Set your general intentions for the day:

....

....

....

....

....

Evening Playbook

GRATITUDE:

List 3 things you are grateful for (which can include future manifestations):

1. ....
....

2. ....
....

3. ....
....

AFFIRMATIONS:

Write 3 affirmations:

1. ....
....

2. ....
....

3. ....
....

FEELINGS:

How did you feel today? ....

How do you feel now? ....

How do you intend to feel tomorrow? ....

INSPIRATION:

Did you receive inspiration today? ....

Describe what you were inspired to do or say ....
....

FOOD EXPERIMENT:

What single item of food did you experiment with today?...........................

Describe how you felt? ....
....

Does your unique body process this food easily? ....

www.ingramcontent.com/pod-product-compliance
Lightning Source LLC
Chambersburg PA
CBHW081824280526
45789CB00007B/2339